TEACHERS!
How Not To Kill the Spirit In Your ADHD Kids

Instead, Understand their Brains
and Turbo-Charge
our Future Leaders & Winners

Sarah Templeton

Gemini Publishing Ltd

Copyright © 2022 Sarah Templeton

The right of the author Sarah Templeton to be identified as the creator of this publication has been asserted. All rights reserved. No part of this publication may be reproduced, distributed, or transmitted in any form or by any means, including photocopying, recording, or other electronic or mechanical methods, without the prior written permission of the publisher, except in the case of brief quotations embodied in critical reviews and certain other non-commercial uses permitted by copyright law.

www.HeadstuffADHDLiberty.co.uk
www.HeadstuffADHDTherapy.co.uk
www.SarahTempleton.org.uk

Illustrations by Sarah Scott Logos and Design

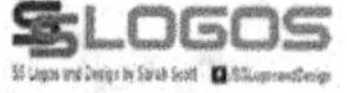

Cover design by Proactive Edge

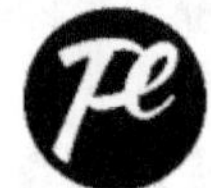

Published 2022
by Gemini Publishing Ltd

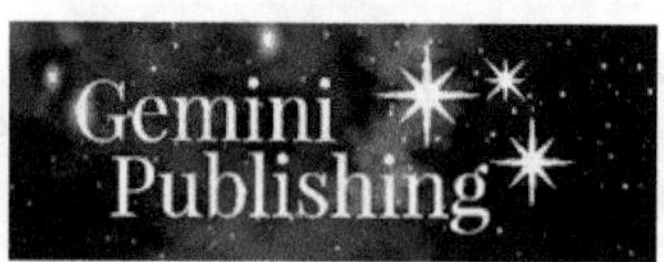

ISBN: 978-1-7399588-2-4

ACKNOWLEDGEMENTS

The first version of this book was written to help parents of ADHD kids. It was called *How Not to Murder Your ADHD Kid: Instead, Learn How To Be YOUR CHILD'S OWN ADHD COACH*, and it only came into existence because of two strong women who, like me, never gave up.

In pole position is Moira, my fantastic tutor at counselling college, who fought more battles for me than any tutor ever should have to. She stuck her neck out for me on more than one occasion to get me through my counselling training which, being undiagnosed ADHD at the time, was torturously tedious and reduced me to tears on many occasions, my short-term memory just not being up to the task of remembering the great paragraphs of corrections I was being asked to do.

But Moira never gave up on me. Even when an unscrupulous supposed 'professional' – working within the prison service – decided to outrightly lie on my college course paperwork, it was Moira who counteracted the whole lot with the awarding body.

She also hollered in the face of this same uncaring person who COULD NOT SEE that all I was trying to do was help young offenders; I sat and sobbed as she stripped me of my prison belt and keys and took me away from my beloved boys.[*] But Moira could see it. She also gave me the best piece of advice, which has stood me in great stead with hundreds of offenders since. 'Always be on their side, Sarah,' she said, 'Always let them know that you are on their side.'

Moira, I will never be able to thank you enough.

Very shortly after I left Moira's college I began with a new counsellor, Lynda. It was Lynda who, on session three, said to me these now famous words, 'Has anybody ever suggested you are

---

[*] Nobody kept me away from my prison boys, though. I wrote to every single one of them, visited them in all the prisons they were shipped out to all over the UK, and I'm still in touch with pretty much all of them to this day.

ADHD?' I was fifty-one. I looked at her with my eyebrows raised and said, 'No! Why?'

'Because I think you are,' she retorted. 'Go home and google it and tell me what you think next week.'

I did and after about 200 lightbulb moments and my entire life dropping into place that night, I tootled off to the NHS – twice – to be told both times that there is no money in the NHS for adult ADHD. I reported this back to Lynda, who was not impressed and told me I should 'go private'.

I saw a private ADHD psychiatrist in London, who told me I couldn't possibly be ADHD because I wasn't diagnosed as a child. On my next session Lynda listened, for about five minutes, as I recounted my experience before exploding, 'I'm sorry but this is bollocks – you are ADHD.' She just wasn't going to accept that I wasn't ADHD and without her firm boot up my bottom I would never have pursued that diagnosis, which has gone on to change my life.

I was diagnosed with not only moderate-to-severe ADHD but three of its comorbidities: severe dyspraxia, dyscalculia and sensory processing disorder. All of these conditions had affected me all my life, but without Lynda being so sure and resolute about getting me diagnosed I would never have reached the understanding of myself that I now have, in my late fifties.

Lynda then went on to be my counselling supervisor for five years as I learnt my ADHD trade, working with hundreds of ADHD kids, adolescents and adults. I learnt more about ADHD from this lady than anyone else. I literally owe her my life. I would never have made sense of my life without her.

This second book has been written purely in response to the thousands of parents across the world who have been thrusting the first book at teachers in a desperate attempt for them to understand their children's brains! So I have hopefully left in all the important stuff but added the best advice I can for teachers and other professionals working with ADHD children and adolescents.

Sarah Templeton, August 2022

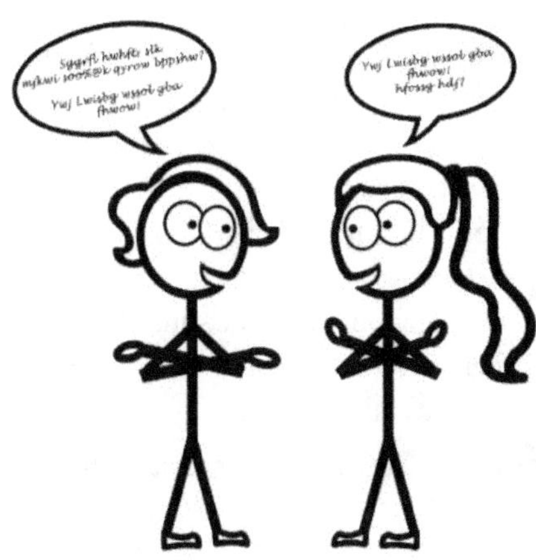

WHAT PROFESSIONALS HAVE SAID ABOUT SARAH TEMPLETON

'I just wanted you to know that the young man we sent you was hugely influenced by his time with you. You changed his whole outlook and attitude to ADHD. He is now very accepting of it and open to the help we are offering him. We could not have done this without your input.'

Andrea Bilbow, The National Attention Deficit Disorder Information and Support Service, ADDISS

'Sarah is an expert in all things ADHD. She works so successfully with ADHD clients because she understands the condition from the inside out.'

Dr Jose Belda, ADHD Psychiatrist

'My son's TEACHER recommended reading Sarah's first book after he and my other son were diagnosed with ADHD. It was so helpful and such an eye opener.'

Parent – on Teacher's Advice

'You won't find another book like this. Written by an experienced counsellor with ADHD who really understands ADHD kids and how to get the best out of them.'

Dr Sawhney, ADHD Specialist Paediatrician

'An extraordinary book! Vital reading for anyone who has an ADHD kid. As a counsellor and psychotherapist I found Sarah's first book fascinating reading from a professional perspective. From a personal perspective I found it extraordinarily moving that Sarah Templeton, who is ADHD, has shared her knowledge and experience from the heart.

'Her passion for supporting and guiding others shines through on every page. Valuable reading for any teacher, counsellor, psychotherapist, doctor or nurse to think about difference and diversity and the needs of ADHD kids and their parents. I would recommend Sarah's books to everyone, regardless of whether or not ADHD has touched your life.'

Head of Counselling, Tutor and Counsellor, Bucks

'Sarah understands ADHD from the inside out and is passionate about turning kids' lives around.'

Dr Helen Read, Psychiatrist, ADHD Consultancy

'I have recommended Sarah a number of times to clients needing ADHD therapy – for her no-nonsense, 'say it as it is' approach.'

Soli Lazarus. B.Ed. (Hons) Psychology, Yellow Sun

'Definitely the 'now what do we do about it?' book we have been all been waiting for!

'Sarah's first book for parents blends insightful knowledge about ADHD with practical strategies that we as parents want to fully understand and accept. It is written and structured in a way that provides help and awareness of ADHD, which moves us forward into manageable situations. We can implement useful help and solutions immediately!

'Sarah clearly shows courage by sharing her own personal experiences and this really strengthens the invisible bond and trust between author and reader. Do get this book today, whether you are a parent or a Life Coach! You will probably never put it out of sight or away on the shelf!'

ADHD/ASD Coach and Qualified Counsellor, Wiltshire

'A MUST for parents of young people with ADHD. As the mother of a teenage boy with extreme ADHD, I cannot recommend Sarah's books enough.

'I love the fact that there are short, sharp chapters for a huge variety of very real problems. I love the no-nonsense, honest advice and strategies, in easy-to-assimilate language. I really love the non-judgmental tone of the author: whether it's the individual stealing, smoking weed, or getting into trouble with the police, she normalises the situation and helps the reader understand what's probably going on and what they might do next.

'And the fact that so many different issues and problems are covered is incredibly valuable and has already helped my family in immeasurable ways. If you are a parent with a child with ADHD, Sarah's first book is what you need to help you on the journey ahead of you. Written by someone who obviously really cares and wants to help young people with ADHD shine, flourish and be happy.'

Accredited Counsellor, Hertfordshire

'Wish this had been written years ago! I have worked with children and young people with ADHD all my adult life. I myself have ADHD as well as both of my children. I have read many, many books about ADHD and I can honestly say, none come close to Sarah's! I wish it had been written sooner. It has really changed my outlook! Cannot recommend it enough!'

Qualified Counsellor, Bedfordshire

'I have referred clients to Sarah and value her professional opinion on clients who I suspect have ADHD. She's never been wrong. Her vast experience in this area has gone a long way to helping people make sense of their lives.'

Accredited Counsellor, Dorset

'Sarah first recognised ADHD in me when I wasn't even there to see her about it! I'm now diagnosed in my mid-40s and as a teacher I am now ADHD-aware enough to spot ADHD in my classroom.

'Sarah 'gets it'. She has been a tremendous help to me personally and professionally and this book will be a great resource for teachers of ADHD children who need a helping hand.'

Suzanne, Headteacher of Infant and Junior School, and mum of two ADHD sons

'Sarah is quite simply The Queen of ADHD! Some medical professionals are qualified up to their armpits and think they know all about ADHD but they really don't. Sarah is qualified, experienced and a walking genius on us ADHDers because she's got it herself.'

Teacher, 32, Berkshire

WHAT READERS THOUGHT OF SARAH'S FIRST BOOK ON PARENTING KIDS:
HOW NOT TO MURDER YOUR ADHD KID – INSTEAD, LEARN HOW TO BE YOUR CHILD'S OWN ADHD COACH

This is an instruction manual on how to manage your ADHD child! AWESOME!

'So I've had lots of different books about ADHD; this is the first book I've read that actually tells me how to help my son. It's been a real game changer. I bought the audiobook as I also have ADHD and struggle to sit and read. My husband listened to it too, which means we are finally on the same page on how to help him and we feel less frustrated.'

Totally understand my son now!

'Thank you so much for this amazing book; everything you have talked about is like you are describing my son! It made me pretty emotional reading it. Now I understand him and what he is going through. I totally recommend this to everyone.'

Loved this book, very informative in a non-patronising way

'Also loved that it is from a UK author as many other books I have read, the authors are American and not as relatable.

Really helped to explain the behaviours of my children and how best to help them. It also concreted the fact that myself and my husband almost certainly are the ones who have passed the ADHD gene on. Would highly recommend this book, I read it in a day and that's great considering my concentration level!'

Gospel according to ADHD

'This book resonated so much with my family. It explains certain behaviour traits for my husband and now my daughter.

Must-have for anyone with ADHD!!'

Buy it! Buy it now!

'This book is a must-buy for anyone who has a child with, or knows anyone with, ADHD. It is so easy to read and/or listen to. Do not hesitate: this will be the best book to help you understand your child/teenager/wife/husband you have ever read and everyone needs to read it! I had to put it down three chapters in because I was feeling so overwhelmed with excitement that somebody 'just got it' Thank you, Sarah, for all your help.'

The ADHD BIBLE! A must-read for parents. Also for adults who may feel they have symptoms.

'This book was lightbulb moment after lightbulb moment. I laughed, I cried, I felt immense relief and clarity when listening.

Now I know why I do what I do, feel how I feel and think how I think. It is THE book to read/hear if you think your child or you yourself as an adult may have symptoms. It makes everything clear and you learn so much more about yourself in a mere few hours. If only I'd known then what I know now.

Thank you, Sarah. You're a genius, who I know is incredibly passionate about helping people with ADHD.

Keep the books coming!'

Practical advice from an experienced author

'I adore everything about this book. It's practically written with advice you can use straightaway as well as some well-researched evidence behind it.

And what could be better than advice from someone who has lived experience? A great book that can be dipped into if you're pushed for time or devoured in a few days.

Highly recommended.'

A revelation

'This book is exceptionally well written and provides amazing insight to my own ADHD tendencies. It has rejuvenated my enthusiasm to engage with and support my son who has been diagnosed at age 8.

I highly recommend.'

Easy to read

'I bought this book and it is amazing, I have read (well, tried to) so many ADHD books but cannot get past first base: I get a major headache. But not with this book. It is such an easy read, I wish I had it years ago. I really do recommend this if your family is living with ADHD. It is a must-read.'

Life-transforming – buy it!

'This is by far and away the BEST book you are going to read on ADHD. Sarah has opened up about so much of her past in an attempt to help parents understand their kids. She's a counsellor with ADHD herself, which is so useful to the reader. She tells us as an adult exactly how her brain worked as a child, which helps us get inside our children's heads.

It's such an easy-to-read book – it was the book title that first grabbed me. Someone who actually understands that although we love our ADHD kids, there are times when I could indeed murder them.

Sarah doesn't beat us up for feeling like that. Instead, she GETS it. She's REAL. She explains things so well – this book is so grounded and practical

Do buy it – no other book on ADHD parenting comes even close to the help you'll get in this one

Thank you Sarah – a true ADHD Angel.'

The best book about ADHD parenting – wise, readable, practical and supportive

'This is a fantastic book for anyone whose child has been diagnosed with ADHD, or who suspects this is the case. Very easy to read, totally grounded in the real world (not in airy, academic theory) and packed with supremely practical, sensible and actionable advice that will help you to avoid emotional meltdowns and be a gentler, savvier parent. Sarah is an absolute 'go-to' expert on this subject. She describes perfectly all the domestic situations encountered regularly by parents with ADHD kids, then takes you inside the mind of your child and gives you strategies to pre-empt or disarm tense situations. If you buy only one book to help you cope, make sure it's this one!'

Easy-to-read and powerful book

'It's very rare I read books that have such an impact on me, but this is one of them. It's such an easy-to-read book (which kind of helps when you have ADHD!). As the title suggests, the book focuses on ADHD in children, but as an adult with potential ADHD I learnt so much about myself, and how to deal with it within the family. There's humour, kindness and a lot of support.'

An absolute godsend!

'This book is AMAZING! I literally read it in one sitting.

Two of my three children have been diagnosed with ADHD and this book has given me such a great understanding of them and their ways. It offers lots of strategies to help and is incredibly informative about the condition.

It's written in such an easy-to-read, relatable format. I recommend you read it if you have ADHD or someone in your life does.'

Really informative, easy to read and VERY useful info!

'I'm working my way through this book and can honestly say it's one of the easiest to follow guides for anyone concerned that a child of theirs might be ADHD. It's set out in such a way that you can choose to just read the bits that you think are most relevant but quite honestly, the author has an excellent writing style so I'm just reading it cover to cover. You can tell that it has been written by someone who really GETS kids with ADHD as opposed to being written by some doctor or other who simply has an opinion on how kids with ADHD should be managed. Fabulous!'

A must-read

'This book is fantastic. Accessible and insightful, what a find. As a parent of a child with ADHD this has given me so much to think about and do to help them with life with ADHD. Books like this should be available in schools and every teacher should read (not a dig at teachers, just in my experience the lack of knowledge of ADHD in schools is frightening). Can't recommend it enough.'

A must-have!

'WOW! Was recommended this book. To begin with I genuinely thought why waste money when I can just look it up online? Oh how WRONG was I. Almost finished the book within one day. It feels like this book was written ABOUT my 6-year-old. Can't thank the author enough. So much information, and it's worded so simply, and really makes you understand what is happening in a child's ADHD brain and why it happens. Honestly this book is worth WAY MORE than it's price tag. Worth Every. Single. Penny. Thank you so much to the author, from a mum who genuinely thought she was at fault and had done something wrong in parenting.'

Finally: a relevant, detailed and down-to-earth resource, that's not American!

'Having pretty much subscribed to all things ADHD that I can find on the internet since last year, I can hand on heart say that this is the most relevant and useful single resource I have acquired to date. Whether you have a diagnosed child, or suspect someone has ADHD in your family, this is the most informative and detailed tool on the market. Sensibly chopped up into meaningful chapters, with real practical solutions and advice for every challenge and scenario that being ADHD can present. Sarah has managed to structure this in a fully engaging way, based on real experiences and tried-and-tested solutions.'

This book saved my family!

'If you are going to buy one book on ADHD this should be it. It is well written by someone who really knows her stuff. It was such a relief to read straightforward advice to what seemed like a very complex situation. The book has educated me so I can now help my son overcome many of the things he was struggling with at home and in school. I have bought four copies of this book so far as I have given copies to my husband, mother and my son's teacher. All of them thought the book was incredibly helpful.'

Awesome

'Picked this up on recommendation to try and understand my 5-year-old daughter. The book was awesome. Informative, very clever and blooming funny to boot. Appealed to my level of humour, was read beautifully on Audible by the author and the techniques I've used from it have already brought my daughter and I closer together and no longer at loggerheads. Thank you.'

A must-read for all ADHD parents!

'Accessible, insightful, bang-on and covers every angle of ADHD imaginable. I read this in 2 days; it made me feel less alone and I was so glad to have better, clearer understanding of ADHD. Sarah Templeton makes it so easy to understand what is going on with these brains!'

Very insightful – a brilliant resource

'This book is a friendly, clear and easy-to-understand resource. It is laid out in easy-to-read chapters which can be referred back to at any point when needed. It's informative, supportive and compassionate. A must-have for anyone looking to understand more about ADHD.'

CONTENTS

BEFORE WE GET GOING A WORD FROM THE AUTHOR — xvii

INTRODUCTION — 1

REALLY IMPORTANT STUFF — 11

THE THREE DIFFERENT TYPES OF ADHD — 14

THE ADHD TRAITS NOBODY TOLD YOU ABOUT — 18

TEACHERS! REALLY IMPORTANT STUFF THAT APPLIES TO ALL ADHD KIDS — 31

WHY ITS UP TO YOU TO SPOT THEIR COMORBIDITIES — 38

THEIR FRAGILE SELF-ESTEEM AND HOW TO HELP THEM HANG ONTO IT — 45

WHEN THEY GET OVERLY EMOTIONAL – EMOTIONAL DYSREGULATION AND REJECTION SENSITIVE DYSPHORIA — 50

WHEN THEY START GETTING INTO TROUBLE WITH TEACHERS — 55

WHEN THEY WON'T STOP FIDGETING AND CAN'T SIT STILL — 66

WHEN THEIR IMPULSIVITY SHOCKS YOU AND THEIR INABILITY TO THINK OF THE CONSEQUENCE DEFIES BELIEF — 70

WHEN YOU CAN'T UNDERSTAND WHY THEY GET SO EASILY DISTRACTED — 75

WHEN INATTENTION CAUSES PROBLEMS — 80

WHEN THEIR FORGETFULNESS IS DRIVING YOU POTTY — 85

WHEN THEIR DISORGANISATION IS CAUSING CHAOS — 90

WHEN THEIR PROCRASTINATION IS WINDING YOU UP — 95

WHEN THEY'RE CONSTANTLY MOANING 'I'M BORED' — 101

SLEEP PROBLEMS AND HOW THEY IMPACT AT SCHOOL — 107

WHEN THEY ALWAYS WANT TO KNOW 'WHY?' — 113

WHEN THEY WON'T DO AS THEY'RE TOLD 117

WHEN THEY ANSWER BACK AND ARGUE WITH YOU 123

WHEN THEY THINK THEY KNOW BEST AND WANT EVERYTHING THEIR OWN WAY 128

WHEN THINGS HAVE TO BE JUST RIGHT – AND PERFECTIONISM 132

WHEN THEY WON'T SHARE 136

WHEN HOMEWORK BECOMES A NIGHTMARE 139

WHEN THEY CAN'T OR WON'T REVISE 147

WHEN HYGIENE GOES OUT THE WINDOW 152

WHEN THEY START GETTING FUSSY ABOUT CLOTHES 156

WHEN FOOD BECOMES A PROBLEM 161

IF THEY START LYING 168

IF YOU FIND OUT THEY ARE STEALING 173

IF YOU SUSPECT OR KNOW THEY ARE USING CANNABIS 178

IF THEY START GETTING IN TROUBLE WITH THE LAW 183

WHAT YOU NEED TO KNOW ABOUT ADHD MEDICATION 195

WHEN YOU ARE ASKED FOR YOUR OPINION ON THERAPY 203

SOME BASIC CBT SKILLS 209

SOME 'AT HOME' SITUATIONS WHICH MIGHT CROSS OVER INTO SCHOOL 215

REWARD SYSTEMS 216

SIBLING RIVALRY 225

WHEN THEY WON'T COME OUT OF THEIR BEDROOM 233

WHEN YOU NEED TO GET THEM OFF GADGETS 236

BEFORE I LET YOU GO 243

WHERE TO FIND MORE ADHD SUPPORT 246

GLOSSARY OF TERMS – WHAT DOES THAT MEAN? 249

WHAT PREVIOUS CLIENTS HAVE SAID ABOUT SARAH 251

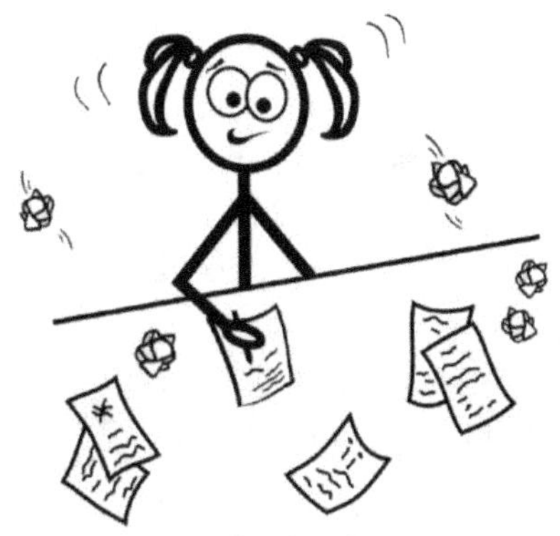

BEFORE WE GET GOING
A WORD FROM THE AUTHOR

Hello.

Welcome to what is hopefully the start of you really understanding just what is going on in your ADHD students' brains. I'm Sarah. I'm a qualified counsellor with an additional qualification in Cognitive Behavioural Therapy (CBT) and I'm also a life coach. My aim with this book is to give as many teachers as possible a THOROUGH understanding of ADHD. My guess is most of you know it is about impulsivity, distraction, inattention and hyperactivity. But how many know about the hundreds of other traits, thoughts and feelings that go alongside ADHD? I certainly knew barely any of them until 2015.

Then, after half a century of exhausting myself, setting up businesses, buying and selling houses and cars, having more ideas per second than most people have in a day, I was finally pounced on by the fifth counsellor I'd seen who said, 'Has anyone ever suggested you have ADHD?'

I looked at her with raised eyebrows. Wasn't ADHD all about nine-year-old boys chucking chairs at teachers? I was a middle-aged counsellor, owner of a highly successful nanny agency and in a ten-year marriage. 'No' I replied. 'Well, I think you are,' she retorted 'so go home and google it.'

I did and, in one evening of increasingly frantic googling, my entire life suddenly dropped into place. It wasn't just one lightbulb moment. It was hundreds. THIS was why I talked too much and over the top of other people. THIS was why I had this horrid internal motor and could not stop working and volunteering. THIS was why nothing ever felt like it was enough, so I was driven to achieve more and more. But it still wasn't enough. THIS was why relaxing or 'just chilling' was alien to me.

It was also why I was bright, quick and became bored so quickly, but could also be gormless when it came to remembering things, dropping things and breaking things. I'd never been able to work out why I was so good at some things and utterly incompetent at others. So many things about me hadn't made sense until that evening.

After a lot of knockbacks from the ill-informed GP's who told me – twice – that there was no money in the NHS for adult ADHD, a private psychiatrist gave my GP a swift kick up the backside and suddenly there WAS money in the NHS! I was referred and diagnosed with moderate-to-severe Combined ADHD within three months.

From that day, in March 2015, my life has revolved around ADHD more than I ever could have imagined. I went on to counsel and coach children, adolescents and adults, both diagnosed with ADHD and those wondering if they have ADHD. I'm an accredited member of the Ayanay Psychological Accreditation organisation and a recognised neurodiversity specialist. I write articles on ADHD and I'm on the All-Party Parliamentary Group for ADHD at the Houses of Parliament. Plus, I trained other counsellors so they could spot ADHD in their therapy rooms.

A very common reason for people coming to see me was parents' lack of understanding of how their ADHD offspring's brains work. The psychiatrists hadn't the time to tell them. The NHS recommends ADHD-specific therapy after diagnosis but then can't afford to provide it. So after their often hard-fought-for diagnosis, usually taking years, parents of ADHD kids are just left dangling with no one to answer their questions – and quite often with some extremely challenging behaviour going on at home and not a clue as to how to deal with it.

And the exact same goes for teachers. Most are desperate to understand and help ADHD kids learn, fit in and enjoy school life. But nobody gave them the handbook!

This is where I come in.

This book aims to give you all the answers to those questions that crop up time after time in my therapy room, and explain how our ADHD different brain wiring gives us a totally different way of seeing things, so subsequently we need different handling to get the best out of us.

I'm going to give you both an insight into how ADHD children think, feel and behave the way they do and, most importantly, the very best way to manage that, using hundreds of tried-and-tested techniques straight from the therapy room and my own ADHD brain!

More than anything, I hope this book helps you have a better understanding of your ADHD students. I hope to give YOU an easier time in the classroom, simple but different ways of doing things, giving THEM a happier childhood. And lessening, if not completely eradicating, the amount of times you get to the end of your tether, storm into the staff room and screech, 'I'm going to bloody murder that little sh*t!!'

Sarah Templeton

Autumn 2022

INTRODUCTION

Oh, not a long introduction that's going to bore me to death! I'm busy!

No. Don't worry; I will keep this bit short, sweet, informative and in easy bite-sized chunks for those of us with short attention spans!

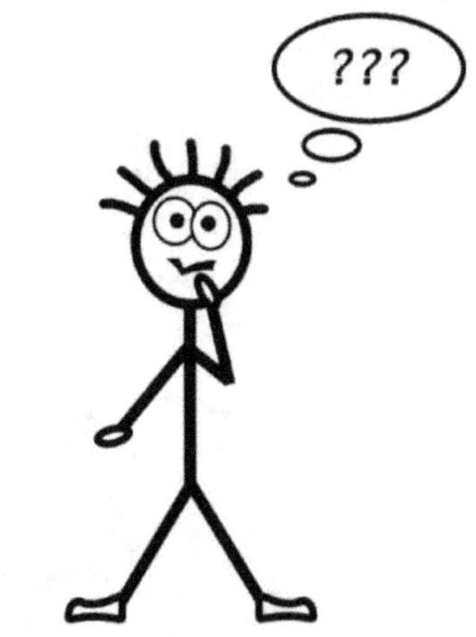

WHO IS THIS BOOK FOR?

Anyone who is working with ADHD kids, whether that's teachers, learning support assistants, SENCOs, social workers, children's services or support workers of any kind. If you are spending ANY time with ADHD children, this book will give you an insider sneaky peek into their brain. It will tell you exactly how their ADHD brain works, how to interact with them successfully and how to get the absolute best out of them in just about every scenario at school but also at home. And definitely, DEFINITELY, make you less inclined to garrotte them!

WHY BOTHER READING IT?

Because it can all go horribly wrong for these kids if you don't. Seriously, not every ADHD kid is going to start smoking weed at nine, get nicked for stealing by ten and be in juvenile court aged eleven. But that can and does happen. I've worked with these adolescents and seen the heart-breaking results of unmanaged ADHD. I'll introduce you to some of these characters throughout the book – not to scare you to death but to inspire you to never, ever give up trying to understand your ADHD students better. A good teacher can change their life. My English teacher did mine. She believed in me enough to tell me, 'You should be a journalist'. I never was but I did finally get my act together enough to write a book!

Young offender units are packed to the rafters with ADHD boys (particularly, but also girls) because nobody took the time to help them use their ADHD to achieve greater things.

So well done YOU for picking up this book. You've already given your current and future students a real fighting chance. I'm in your corner. Stick with me and together we will give your ADHD students the absolute best start in life there is.

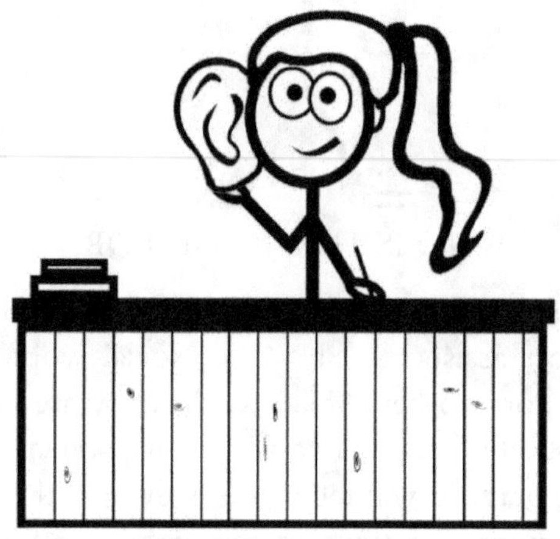

WHY SHOULD YOU LISTEN TO ME?

Because I get it. I really, REALLY, get it. Diagnosed moderate-to-severe ADHD myself, I'd spent fifty years not knowing I had any disorder at all. Yes, I thought differently, spoke faster, did things the quick way and always seemed out of kilter with normal, dare I say, 'boring' people! But I had zero clue that this was because I had any kind of condition. I had never been known as a SEND kid, nor come into contact with mental health services. Why would I? I honestly believed I was the one getting it right, and everybody else was dragging their heels behind!

Then I began work in the English prison system. Back then, I didn't know I was ADHD. All I knew was that I totally GOT these boys, their low boredom thresholds, their need for thrills and excitement, their loathing of authority and their belief that they were always right. I described the way I bonded with each and every offender who slouched in front of me in a grey prison-issue tracksuit, as 'magical'.

Then came that lightbulb moment: my own diagnosis. Only THEN did I realise I got them because they were all like me: ADHD. On further inspection, I discovered that roughly 50% of the young offenders I was working with had been diagnosed ADHD as children, but the rest had no clue. Just like me. They knew they felt and thought differently to 'normal people' but were perplexed as to why.

Since then I have worked with thousands of young offenders and adolescent ADHD kids who have been getting into trouble with the law. I recognise their strong drive for excitement and adrenaline and can understand all that they do and still respect them. I encourage them to see that they CAN have all the excitement they need without any involvement in drugs, alcohol or crime, and now I'm proud to say I count many of Britain's young offenders as some of my best friends.

It is my deepest joy when I turn another ADHD youngster away from the court and prison system and give them back their freedom and the right to choose the life they want.

But before it gets to this point, it all starts back at school. Which is why I have written this book. The more you understand ADHD kids' brains, the less they are going to have to kick against. Work WITH your ADHD students. The more understanding and support they have from you, with the help of this book, the less likely they are going to find themselves up in front of any judge. Your ADHD students need to know that you are on their side, that you are doing your damnedest to understand them and that together you can not only get to grips with their ADHD, but also put them on the path to a hugely successful life.

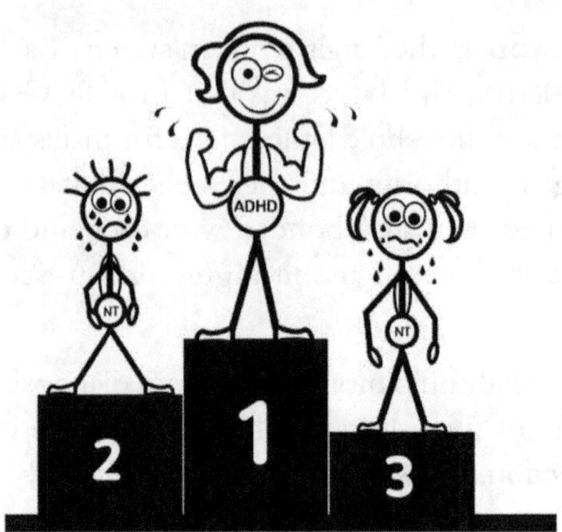

SO WHATS ALL THIS ABOUT LEADERS AND WINNERS?

Well it might come as a big surprise to you, but it's true!

Until you found this book you might have assumed that ADHD kids, along with other special educational needs and disabilities (SEND) kids, would have trouble succeeding in life after they leave school. But I have very good news for you – and them! Tons of ADHD kids DO become our leaders and winners. The reasons for this will become apparent throughout the book but for now let me just tell you:

- ADHD people have more drive than other people

- They don't like coming second

- They are constantly looking for something new and exciting

- Those who are 'the clown of the class' often go on to become comedians, entertainers, actors and performers

- They have more compassion than others, so do great things in the caring professions

- They get bored easily, so very few ADHD people only have one job. They say all entrepreneurs have ADHD – and if not all, then it's definitely most.

- They are adrenaline seekers, so most of Hollywood's stuntmen and women are ADHD.

- They are extremely competitive, so a lot of Olympians, world record holders and elite sports people are ADHD.

- They have a heightened sense of justice and feel strongly about what is right and wrong so a lot of them end up in politics, heading up charities and changing the world.

So instead of seeing that kid who won't sit still and is constantly restless as an irritating little toad, try thinking of him at the Olympics in eight years.

And the kid who won't stop talking, distracting others and making people laugh, he will probably be on a one-man stadium tour with his comedy show in ten years' time.

The boy who won't stop climbing trees, jumping on the school roof and getting himself into all sorts of dangerous situations, he could be working in Hollywood as a stuntman.

That little girl who always thinks she's right, will argue the toss about anything and can convince everybody her way is the only way, she's going to end up in the Houses of Parliament.

The constantly distracted, dreamy and 'in her own world' girl could be our next Poet Laureate.

ADHD people don't walk the middle line. You won't find many who have worked at the council for thirty years! You will find a huge amount of very successful ADHD people in every field you can think of but there are some, who don't have the right support or anything even close to it, who do end up going down the adrenaline-seeking criminal path. Sadly, the young offender units and adult prisons are full of these ADHD adrenaline-seekers purely because they haven't had the right assessment, diagnosis and medication and I am particularly passionate about this group. Because they could be just as successful as the rest if they only received the right attention from an early age and the right medical, family and school support.

You only have to google 'successful ADHD people' to see a list as long as your arm, but some who have been very out and proud about their ADHD diagnosis are:

- Tom Hanks – Actor, Film Maker

- will.i.am – Singer, Songwriter, Record Producer
- Whoopie Goldberg – Actor, Comedian, Author
- Rob Beckett – Comedian, TV Presenter
- Russell Brand – Comedian, Actor, Activist
- Lee Mack – Comedian, Actor, TV Presenter
- Anthony McPartlin – TV Presenter, Singer, Comedian
- Will Smith – Actor, Singer, Producer
- Justin Bieber – Singer, Songwriter
- Lewis Hamilton – Formula One Champion
- Channing Tatum – Actor, Playwright
- Justin Timberlake – Singer, Songwriter, Record Producer, Actor
- Melanie Brown, The Spice Girls – Singer, Songwriter
- Cher – Singer, Actor
- Cameron Diaz – Actor, Author
- Bill Gates – Founder of Microsoft
- Kurt Cobain, Nirvana – Singer, Songwriter
- Jamie Oliver – Chef, TV Presenter, Restaurateur
- Britney Spears – Singer, Actor
- Michael Phelps – Most decorated Olympian of all time

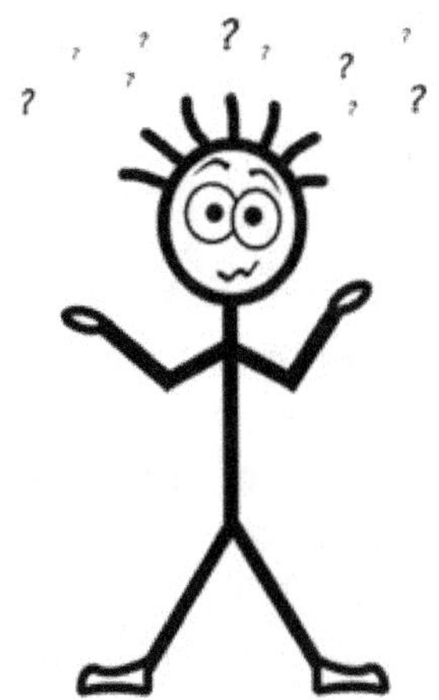

SO HOW WILL THIS BOOK HELP?

Hopefully in a big way! Because that is my aim. Firstly a HUGE THANKS from me right now and – in advance – from all the ADHD kids you will be helping in future by reading this book.

I'm guessing you've picked up this edition because you are either a teacher or a learning support assistant in a school – maybe in a school for kids with special educational needs. Perhaps you work with children professionally in another capacity and are enlightened enough to know that a lot of these kids will have either undiagnosed or diagnosed ADHD.

Whichever way it is, if you are coming into contact with ADHD children, I am genuinely so grateful that you are interested enough in their wellbeing to have decided to read this book.

Teachers are in a unique position to spot not only undiagnosed ADHD but all of its 'comorbidities' or coexisting conditions. Sadly, as I write in 2022, I know that ADHD and neurodiversity barely feature in teacher training and this is something we are passionate about changing.

But please don't think there is any judging going on from me that you haven't been trained in how to spot or work with ADHD. It's a large, gaping hole in teaching training and, until that gap is filled, I'll do my very best, in this book, to give you every scrap of information you need to help identify and work with ADHD in your students, to give those children the best chance of being happy and successful at school.

I'd like to give you my own example of how critical and pivotal your role is in children receiving the right education.

I was a reasonably bright child at junior school coming in the top one third of the class at exam time. When I took the 12+ (which was a test paper full of 'problems'), my undiagnosed ADHD, coupled with my undiagnosed dyscalculia, meant I looked at these problems and my brain didn't have a clue how to work them out. It's not that I didn't want to: my brain just didn't work that way. And it wasn't until I was fifty-five years old and diagnosed with dyscalculia that we worked out WHY my brain didn't work that way. People with dyscalculia cannot work out problems.

Anyway back to my tragic tale.

The results were in and although 50% of my class of thirty-one had passed, which meant I should have been safely within that top half, I had failed.

My headmaster appealed before the results were even sent to parents, to try and get me into the grammar school, but was turned down. When the results were publicly released, my mother again appealed but the education authority told her that because I had failed 'so spectacularly' they couldn't possibly put me through to the grammar school. My headmaster was incensed, ranting, 'If she'd been given an English, maths and French test, she'd have sailed through.'

Fast forward a year to the end of year exams at my grotty secondary modern school, and I came first in English and first in maths out of 132 students. The headmistress rang my mother and told her that I 'shouldn't be at this school' and she 'had secured a place for me at the grammar school'. I didn't find this out until I was sixteen because when my mother had been sent the grammar school uniform list, she simply couldn't afford to buy a complete new school uniform when she had done so the year before.

So I spent four years at a school I shouldn't have been at, where I was bored rigid and not stretched or pushed to achieve my potential, purely because nobody had spotted my ADHD and my dyscalculia.

This was in the mid-1970s. It would be wonderful to say, 'Well thank goodness that doesn't happen anymore,' but tragically it's STILL happening every day in our schools. ADHD and its comorbidities are being missed just as much today as they were fifty years ago. This makes me sad and angry in equal measures.

But YOU are in the very best position possible to make sure this doesn't happen to other kids.

I am going to help YOU change other kids' lives so they don't end up like me: bitter, angry, resentful and annoyed that nobody spotted these conditions in me when they were pretty obvious!

HOW though?

I'm going to break it down for you. There will be no sweeping generalisations. I will be going into every ADHD trait and idiosyncrasy, most of which I have myself and all of which I have worked with over the years. By the time you get to the end of this book you will be able to pick up indicators of ADHD in your students and, by doing so, change their lives for the better.

Each chapter will explain a different trait, exactly what is going on in the child's brain and how that will be playing out at school, with different strategies for managing the behaviour.

Some of you may be teachers AND parents of ADHD kids. So the helpful-at-home stuff has been left in from my first book, which was written for parents. This will also give non-ADHD-parent teachers an insight into just what parents have to deal with at home, and illustrate why sending parents on a standard 'parenting course' really isn't going to be of much use here!

The book is structured in such a way that you can dip in and out, just reading the bits that relate to your particular ADHD student/s – and any confusing, challenging or perplexing behaviours they are presenting in the classroom – right now.

There are places for notes and a summary at the end of each section so if you are literally at screaming point and need a one-sentence refresher on what is really going on in the ADHD child's brain, you can grab the book quickly and have an immediate answer as to how you should handle the current situation as it's happening.

I wish you the very best of luck. And please always remember that your ADHD students are extremely lucky to have you. Why? Because by picking up this book you've already shown you are trying to understand them. Remember, nobody EVER tried to understand me, nor tens of thousands of other ADHD adults who are only just getting diagnosed.

The fact that you really want to understand their ADHD is huge for any ADHD child. So give yourself a big pat on the back and let's get started.

REALLY IMPORTANT STUFF

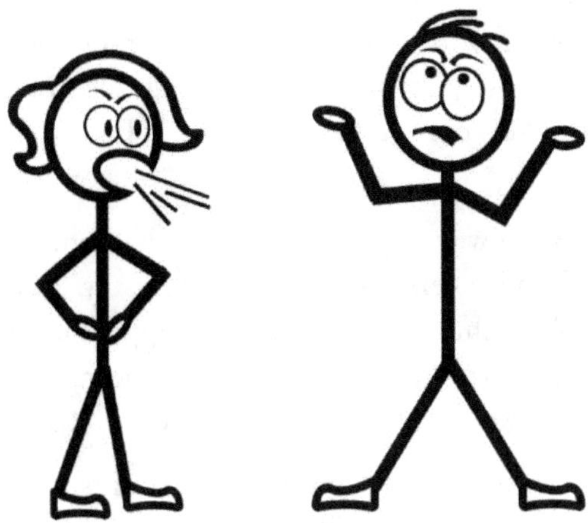

WHY IT'S IMPORTANT WE GET THE PARENTS SORTED TOO

I bet your first thought is, 'Well this has got nothing to do with me'.

But actually it has. Because if you have an ADHD child in your class then odds are at least one if not both their parents are ADHD as well. And the odds are even higher that they won't know it! They probably won't know that the condition is hugely inheritable and the current reckoning is ADHD is likely to be inherited by 85% of children who have at least one parent with it. It is now accepted ADHD is as inheritable as eye colour and height.

ADHD adults are also attracted to each other so there's often a chance both parents will have it.

And if you have one or two parents with undiagnosed ADHD and a child/children also undiagnosed, I can't begin to tell you the clashes that causes at home. It's not going to be harmonious, put it that way!

How parents interact with their ADHD child will be majorly affected by whether they are ADHD themselves or not. Just because their ten-year-old is punching walls and kicking his brother and they wouldn't DREAM of such behaviour, doesn't necessarily mean they aren't ADHD themselves.

I can't begin to tell you how many of the hundreds of ADHD parent clients I've worked with who have casually mentioned, 'Well I've never been able to sit still and I've always been a terrible sleeper/overthinker/compulsive drinker but I've never been as bad as HIM!'

Those parents are always shocked to know that while ADHD is most often inherited, the severity and impact of it isn't. So their tearaway teen may well be exhibiting off-the-scale appalling behaviour, the like of which they would NEVER think of doing themselves, but that does not necessarily mean they are not also ADHD.

I have also lost count of the number of parents who believe that just because their child 'is just like me' they can't have ADHD, when in fact the parents are as ADHD as the child. They just haven't noticed anything different because there is nothing different. They are both displaying ADHD traits without even realising it.

If you are working with parents to better understand their ADHD child, you could help them identify the source of the ADHD by very gently, and of course sensitively, finding out if anybody in the immediate or past family:

- Has had long-term anxiety or depression

- Has addiction problems

- Are workaholics

- Have been in prison

- Are often angry or violent

- Struggle with their weight

- Are always on the go

- Has been diagnosed with another mental health problem like bipolar disorder or emotionally unstable personality disorder

Chances are higher it is these family members who have undiagnosed ADHD. This can be quite a shocking revelation to a lot of parents so it does need to be handled extremely sensitively. But you will be doing them a huge favour if you are able to guide them in the direction of the correct diagnosis and medication for themselves, as this will have a very direct and positive effect on their child.

Another good reason for helping parents understand they might have the condition is because it will help the younger ADHD members of the family not feel so alone with their ADHD, if they know that Mum/Dad/Brother/Aunt Flo are also ADHD tribe members. I've seen the look of relief on dozens of kids' faces when they realise it isn't just them.

So it is well worth gently nudging parents to find out where the ADHD has come from.

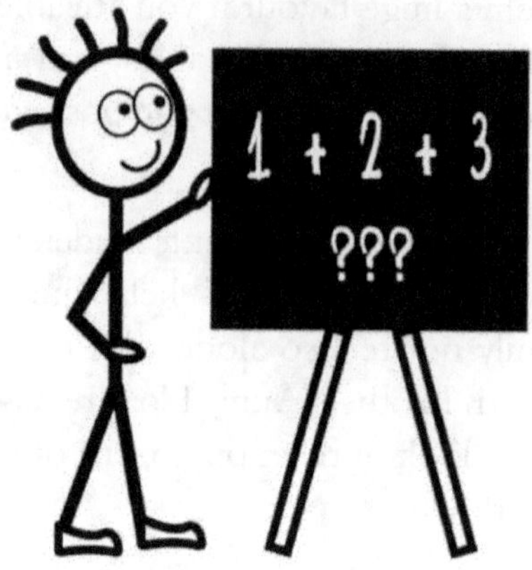

THE THREE DIFFERENT TYPES OF ADHD

I find it incredibly strange that more and more paediatricians and psychiatrists are diagnosing both children and adults purely as 'ADHD' without going into any detail of which variation of the condition they have.

When I was diagnosed back in early 2015, I was told which type and its severity. This was common in those days. You were told whether you had Hyperactive/Impulsive ADHD, Inattentive ADHD or Combined, which is a combination of the two. You were told also whether your ADHD was mild, mild-to-moderate, moderate, moderate-to-severe or severe. I don't know why they have stopped diagnosing this way, but most clients now are coming into therapy with a diagnosis of ADHD, plain and simple. This really is not helpful to either the child with the condition, or their parents, family or teachers. There is such a huge difference in the types and varying severity of them, and the first thing you really need to do is find out which category every ADHD student falls into. If the child's diagnoser has been a bit sketchy with the info, read on.

Hyperactive/Impulsive ADHD: this category, applied traditionally to boys, means they have endless energy and do things very impulsively. If you think about nine-year-old boys who are constantly fighting, tearing about, have grazes on their knees, get stuck up trees and throw chairs at teachers, this is your archetypal

Hyperactive/Impulsive ADHD child. They are also typically loud, talkative, argumentative, think they know best about everything, very fidgety, unable to sit still and are generally demanding and IN YOUR FACE!

The polar opposite of this is Inattentive ADHD, which traditionally was thought to affect mainly girls. If you think about when you were at school, or your students now, there is usually at least one girl who is the daydreamer, the one who seems to be 'away with the fairies' or 'always in her own world'. She (or we now know, just as possibly HE) is usually very sweet and kind and everybody likes them but they are known for being very dreamy. This is your traditional Inattentive ADHD child. These kids share a lot of traits with the Hyperactive/Impulsive and Combined category, but most often they don't show it. Their restlessness and hyperactivity is all in their mind. They still have busy brains with lots of thoughts, but they don't show them or put them into action like the other two categories.

Those with Inattentive ADHD usually struggle hugely with a lack of motivation and chronic procrastination. They have a lot of ideas which are very rarely put into practice because they don't have the motivation to follow through and complete tasks. They tend to end up feeling like underachievers because they've had plenty of ideas, hopes and dreams but very seldom fulfil them. Those with this kind of ADHD usually present as very quiet. They don't speak a lot, especially in groups. They come across as calm and sensible, but inside their brains, it is a different matter. They struggle with distraction a lot as well and focus is a real problem for them. These ADHD kids are always going to be harder for you to spot as they blend into the background more.

Then you've got the biggest category of all (and this is the one I am in): the 'Combineds'. This group, as I always say, have got it all going on! We are hyperactive/Impulsive, have racing brains, can't sit still, are always on the go, always wanting the next thing, say and do things impulsively and can be quite obnoxious! But we also have problems with distraction, inattention, brain fog and a degree of lack of motivation, along with procrastination when it comes to things which are boring or dull and don't stimulate our brains.

As time has moved on, we now know boys can have Inattentive ADHD – and it is now reasonably commonplace. Girls can have purely Hyperactive/Impulsive ADHD – but much less so in my experience.

Teaching these three different types of ADHD quite obviously needs to be very different. If you have an Inattentive child, it is their lack of motivation, their procrastination and their inability to focus and concentrate that's going to give you the biggest problems. If it's a Hyperactive/Impulsive or Combined child you're going to have to deal with most of those traits but also an incredible restlessness; always wanting to move, always wanting to do the next thing and usually more attitude and anger.

The severity of the impact on them also matters hugely. If you have a child with mild or mild-to-moderate traits you aren't going to have too much to deal with. Probably lack of concentration in class will be a problem and you might find them difficult to motivate because of procrastination. But you also probably won't be dealing with an awful lot of the other traits people diagnosed moderate or severe will be displaying. It is the moderate-to-severe and severely impacted ADHD people who really struggle at school and in life. Their traits impact them to the point that life becomes difficult and your teaching skills will be tested to the limit!

Worry not. Help is at hand in this book!

TOP TEACHING TIPS … Know which ADHD type your students have. And have a good read up on it. Know which traits are likely to be impacting them more because of the type of ADHD they have.

WHAT WORKS BEST … Not assuming all people with ADHD are the same – that couldn't be further from the truth. Understand that no two ADHD people are the same. They all have different traits, all with different severities and nearly always with different comorbidities.

Important stuff I want to remember:

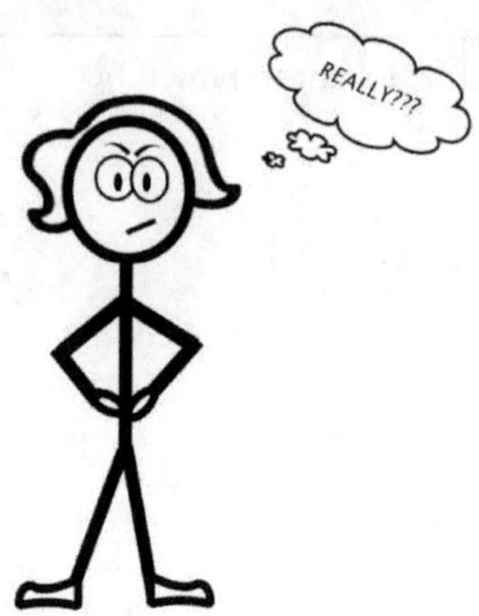

THE ADHD TRAITS NOBODY TOLD YOU ABOUT

Read this bit BEFORE you go further, as this section alone might help you understand why ADHD children think/do/say SO MUCH stuff that presses your buttons.

ADHD isn't all about inattention, distraction, impulsivity and hyperactivity. In fact, that's only a very small part of ADHD in my view. It is these traits HERE that will have a daily impact in your classroom but once you understand this is how an ADHD brain works, dealing with and managing behaviour will become a whole lot easier. So … Deep breath, and off we go.

ADDICTION

ADHD people are at a much higher risk of developing addiction issues. And we aren't just talking alcohol and drugs, although they often feature heavily in undiagnosed teens and adults. The ADHD brain loves excitement, the buzz, adrenaline and when it GETS it, it LIKES it SO MUCH it wants more! Look out for the first signs of this in ADHD children. Addiction can start young. But is not to be confused with fixation. More on that later.

The ADHD brain loves sweet things so if cakes, biscuits, chocolate or sweeties start being consumed in noticeable quantities and the child's waistline is expanding at the same time, you can be pretty sure a sugar addiction is on the way.

ADHD brains are also compulsive, as well as impulsive. So once the brain gets a taste for that yummy sweetness it is going to want more, and more and more!

Other addictive behaviour often seen in ADHD kids is gaming, shopping, gambling and, especially with boys, cannabis smoking.

ADRENALINE JUNKIES

The ADHD brain craves adrenaline. Because in simple non-scientific terms (I couldn't stand my science teacher – you'll see the relevance of that later) the brain doesn't have enough dopamine, which is the pleasure 'everything's enough' hormone. So in the ADHD brain, there's just not enough excitement going on. This is why an eight-year-old may have flung himself off the school roof. Or climbed a tree so high he got stuck. He will be doing it, unknowingly, for the buzz. Feeding his adrenaline-seeking brain.

ALWAYS KNOWING BEST

This is one of the traits that causes the most trouble. We do always think we know best. My theory on this is that our brains work quicker than neurotypicals, so we can usually think of a quicker, easier way of doing things. We can't see any reason why anyone else wouldn't want things done our way too.

BEST IN A CRISIS

This is an interesting trait. When there is a crisis such as a car accident, it is the ADHD person who will react quickest and most calmly. And that's because when ADHD brains get flooded with adrenaline they can focus, concentrate and take action much more swiftly than when things are 'normal'. That's why ADHD adults make fantastic paramedics.

CLEANLINESS

Or lack of. Most ADHD kids go through a patch of not wanting to have a shower or a bath, or clean their teeth. I certainly did. I remember going to the dentist once and having to have four fillings because I had decided that cleaning my teeth was way too boring so I'd given it up several weeks before. Around the same age, twelve-ish, I decided that bathing was also a waste of my valuable time, so I used to run a bath and sit next to it on a stool reading my book and swishing my fingers in the water every few minutes to fool my mother. I've even met ADHD adults who can't be bothered with the whole 'cleaning yourself' palaver, so if any of your students go through this anti-washing period, don't be surprised.

CLUMSINESS

ADHD kids are usually clumsy, and this often carries through to adulthood. We drop things, break things and damage things on a regular basis. This is caused by a combo of doing things too quickly, not concentrating, getting distracted and being inattentive. 'If anyone's going to knock it over, it'll be you' regularly rang in my ears when I was young and had yet again collided with a mug of tea nestling by someone's ankles.

COMPASSIONATE

This is much less known about ADHD but very true. We have more compassion than most. It is why so many ADHD adults give up their time volunteering or working with people or animals in need. We care, usually deeply, and seeing suffering hurts us.

COMPULSIVITY

The ADHD brain is very powerful. If it finds something it likes – from biscuits to bungee jumping – it is going to demand more and more. And it won't let you stop. Ask any ADHD person if they can stop at one of anything. The likelihood is they can't.

DIFFICULTY INTERPRETING INSTRUCTIONS AND DIRECTIONS

This is a trait that is much lesser known but one that has a big impact, especially at school. ADHD brains see or take things differently, and this includes how they interpret instructions and directions from teachers. Sometimes we just haven't got a clue what the teacher actually MEANS until we see somebody else doing it. The ADHD child might not even know this is a problem. Throughout my school years I certainly didn't. But I did know that I often had to glance over the shoulder of the person sitting next to me to understand what the teacher meant. As soon as I glimpsed them starting the work, I knew what I was supposed to be doing. Be very careful about this one because if a child is angry, rude or refusing to do work at school this COULD be the reason behind it.

EMOTIONAL DYSREGULATION

Now here's a biggie. In simple terms this means we can't regulate our emotions. Because the executive function part of the ADHD brain that controls emotions doesn't work. What this actually means is an ADHD person's emotions can be all over the place. We can be literally feeling perfectly happy one moment, then a wave of misery can sweep over us. Then ten minutes later be happy as Larry again. This is confusing for teachers and carers, but even more unnerving for the person going through it.

To give you an idea of how impactful this trait is, in the last few years it is been agreed by psychiatrists in the field that the biggest impact of ADHD on someone is not the hyperactivity, distraction, impulsivity or inattention. It is the emotional dysregulation, the inability to react appropriately to emotions.

ADHD people can't regulate their emotions. They might laugh at funerals or cry at TV adverts. They will often get called 'over sensitive', or 'drama queen'. Any ADHD person you talk to will admit this is one of the most difficult aspects of the condition.

EXCESSIVE TALKING AND TALKING OVER PEOPLE

This one makes us very unpopular! While Inattentive ADHD people are often quiet and withdrawn, your Combineds and Hyperactives rarely shut up! Our brains are going full speed and we can't get the words out of our mouths quick enough.

ADHD people speak over others and interrupt primarily because if they don't say their thought immediately, it'll be forgotten. Our short-term memory is so poor, we can't hold a thought long enough for you to finish speaking.

FIXATIONS

Once the ADHD brain has found something it likes, it can get extremely fixated or obsessed with it. With children this is often one toy, one teddy or one doll. As they get older it can be one computer game, one sport or one love interest. With an ADHD brain, it is all-or-nothing. We either LOVE something with a passion or it is boring and we are over it!

HEIGHTENED SENSE OF JUSTICE

Another unusual one. But this will explain why an ADHD student is often heard wailing, 'But it is NOT fair.' This would seem to be a bit of a contradiction. After all, aren't ADHD peeps the ones who break rules and loathe authority? Yep. But those same people have a very strong sense of what is right and fair. We hate injustice, discrimination, being ripped off or anyone being taken advantage of. And we won't keep quiet about it.

HYPER FOCUS

Generally thought to be when the normally chaotic and busy brain finds something it really likes. So much so, it banishes all the cluttered thinking, enabling it to concentrate solely on this one exciting new thing. For example, a new interest, like rugby. An ADHD kid won't do anything by halves. If they've decided rugby is their new 'thing' they will eat, sleep and breathe it. They will want every piece of new kit, beg to be taken to rugby matches, be YouTubing it till all hours and admonishing Mum for 'ruining their life' if she refuses to sign them up to a pricey rugby academy. Then, when they've whinged about it till everyone's ears bleed, they'll get bored and decide football is much more their thing!

LABELS IN CLOTHES

Ask the next person you meet to show you the back of their jumper. If the label's been snipped, or torn off in anger, odds are that's an ADHD person who cannot STAND the itchiness of labels. The first thing I do when I arrive home from shopping is grab the scissors and cut out every label, washing instruction and those especially annoying hanger loops! Even the thought of labels is making me itch.

LOSING THINGS

This is one of the biggest frustrations both for and with ADHD kids. From school jumpers to pens, PE kits to text books, and – at home – especially the TV remote! We just cannot find ANYTHING. And I can tell you why. It is because we can't remember where we put it. And why is that? The first ADHD psychiatrist I ever met told me this gem. 'For a thought to be stored as a memory, it has to be thought for so many millionths of a second. And an ADHD brain rarely thinks a thought for long enough.' So we literally don't think the thought, 'I'm putting my pen in my pencil case' long enough for it to become a memory. So have patience with kids on this one. They'll need visual reminders of where things are.

LYING

Why do ADHD kids lie? Not all of them will – but a big chunk do. And I include myself in that. I started lying around twelve-ish. Nothing criminal, apart from the odd swipe of chocolate from the newsagent. It was more to do with spicing up my life. One classic was when I'd been late into school after a GP visit. I was later back than expected so told the whole class it was because a male patient had dropped dead in the waiting room. Lord knows why I chose that. And I was found out later the very same day when someone mentioned it to my mother.

There are different theories on why ADHD kids lie. My own is that it makes life more dramatic and therefore interesting. And we do hate boring! Also, we have very poor short-term memory, so sometimes what we genuinely think is the truth, actually isn't. Then there's the need for thrills and excitement. I remember vividly scrawling swear words all over my library book, aged about thirteen. My mother hauled me in front of the chief librarian to apologise – indignant that it WAS NOT ME – and berated the librarian, who really should have taken MUCH MORE CARE before releasing books with this FILTH all over them. I remember that poor woman's blushing face to this day – and I still feel guilty.

MELTDOWNS

I bet some of you have come to this section first! The clever people will tell you (probably the ones who liked their science teacher) that meltdowns are because the ADHD brain gets overloaded with emotion and doesn't know how to cope. I will tell you that ADHD meltdowns are usually because the child is feeling frustrated, angry, not understood, that something isn't fair or a multitude of other reasons why things are not going their way.

MUDDLING WORDS UP

This is a less known trait but one that seems to affect us all. Our brain doesn't seem to be able to recall the actual word we want. So for example I will often use the word 'cushion' when I mean 'pillow' or the word 'glass' when I mean 'window'.

NO RESPECT FOR AUTHORITY

Here we go! This is a humdinger of a trait; it is the one that gets boys locked up in prison and the one that gets us into trouble at school. And as we get older it is the one that gets us into trouble at work. It is also the reason why a massive percentage of adult ADHD people are self-employed. Because, put simply, we do not like being told what to do! There is a caveat here. If we respect somebody, for example a particular teacher (and nearly always this is because they treat us with respect) we will normally be putty in their hands. But anybody who talks down to us, who is overly authoritative or tells us what to do in anything other than a kind and encouraging manner, beware. It presses the wrong buttons in us and you'll often get a verbal, or even physical, negative reaction.

NOTHING EVER BEING ENOUGH

We have the ADHD brain to thank for this one as well. It is that lack of dopamine, which means we are never satisfied; whatever it is we are doing it is usually not enough. The ADHD brain always wants more. More food, more drink, to stay up later, to stay on a computer game longer. It is never satisfied and always wants more.

NOT THINKING OF THE CONSEQUENCE

ADHD brains don't have the ability to do this. And it is one of the main reasons young offender units are packed with ADHD teens. I'll give you an example of how severe this trait is. I was trying stimulant meds for the first time and threw my house keys down on the edge of a small table. I glanced back at them and thought, 'Don't leave them there; if they fall down the back you won't know where they've gone.' I then stood rooted to the spot, in shock. Proper shock. I realised that was the FIRST TIME I had EVER thought of a consequence. Of anything. In over half a century! I'd had no idea before this that my brain wasn't giving a thought to any consequence. Ever.

Give this trait a lot of thought. It is a serious issue for ADHD kids. When you want to holler at them, 'WHY in God's name didn't you THINK before you … (insert any number of careless, hapless, dangerous activities)?' Their answer should be, 'Because my brain didn't think of the consequence.' It won't be, though, because they won't be aware of it. It is up to the adult to understand this and work with them to try to think before they speak/act because there's little hope of it happening naturally.

OVERWHELM

This is a very little known trait but every ADHD adult you talk to will know this plays a big part in how they feel at times. And ADHD kids have it too. They just won't know how to name the feeling. ADHD brains are unusual in that they can go from feeling everything is okay one minute to being totally overwhelmed the next, without any gradual build-up. Thankfully the converse is true and the intense feeling of overwhelm and not being able to cope can pass just as quickly. But it is debilitating and the effect of it shouldn't be underestimated. I've sold off properties at great financial loss because the feelings of overwhelm were too much to bear. And kids will definitely kick-off at school if they are overwhelmed.

POOR CONCEPT OF TIME

This is a strange one but one that everybody with ADHD has. We have a very poor concept of ALL time. That includes time in the past, the present and the future. In the past we find it very difficult to know how long ago something was. A simple question like, 'When did you last do any maths homework?' is likely to be met by a blank face and an, 'I don't know.' This is not an ADHD child being deliberately vague. They probably have no clue.

Time issues in the present mean we are very poor judges of how long something is going to take. Neurotypical kids can work out that tidying up their room, packing their schoolbag and having a shower before tea will take forty minutes. The ADHD kid will tell you fifteen – and mean it. I was shocked to find out only recently I had a reputation for being late. Then I realised I had hardly any idea how to work out how long anything was going to take. It is always just a random guess.

PROCRASTINATION

Now this is a huge one. And very probably the trait that could potentially be giving you more problems with your ADHD students than any other. Procrastination is a strange one when it comes to ADHD. Those of us who are Combined or Hyperactive often don't have much trouble with it. Our problem is more often not being able to do things quickly enough. But people with Inattentive ADHD and Combined ADHD who are high on the Inattentive side, can have absolutely colossal problems with procrastination. Procrastination is also the reason why people with ADHD are often called 'lazy'. They are far from it actually, but it can present as chronic laziness.

It is an executive malfunction in the ADHD brain that is responsible for procrastination problems. You might have heard the expression 'brain fog'. A lot of people with ADHD describe their brain as if it is surrounded by thick cotton wool or doing anything at all is like walking through treacle and they can't get it to move or function in any way. A lot of ADHD people know exactly what needs doing and how to do it, but they cannot get their brain to propel them into doing it. This goes for adults too. Medication can help hugely with procrastination, but until a child is on the right dose of the right medication you may find their procrastination and inability to just get on with things, will drive you round the twist.

The scientific explanation for this is that an ADHD brain will only get motivated by something it finds exciting. So you can bet your life if their parents are offering pizza, chips and ice cream, an ADHD child won't find it hard to find the motivation to sit at the dinner table. It is when asking them to do their homework that the procrastination will kick in. It is really not them being difficult, although this is how it will seem. The brain is a powerful driver and unless there is excitement and adrenaline involved, an ADHD brain will put off doing whatever is dull and repetitive or lacking in excitement.

PUSHING BOUNDARIES

This is a trait that has a very big impact, especially on teenagers. It goes along with thinking we know best and wanting things our own way. ADHD people on the whole have very little respect for boundaries and want to push against all of them. Ironically ADHD kids AND adults work better in a structured environment, but expect ADHD children to kick against boundaries. Our brain just doesn't like being told what to do.

REJECTION SENSITIVE DYSPHORIA (RSD)

This is something very few people know about, but it will almost definitely have a huge impact on all ADHD children, especially when they hit puberty. Rejection sensitive dysphoria quite literally means an out-of-proportion oversensitivity to rejection. In literal terms this will mean that ADHD children are very sensitive to rejection, in particular humiliation or criticism. And they will often react to rejection with anger, either verbal or physical. RSD also means an ADHD brain will perceive rejection when it is not really there. Perceived rejection can be as cripplingly painful as actual rejection. Their reaction to it often leads them to be called drama queens, or labelled as overly sensitive, and accusations of always wanting to be the centre of attention.

RISK-TAKING AND THRILL-SEEKING

This is a trait that can often take ADHD people in one of two directions. The need for adrenaline and excitement can mean a lot of ADHD people engage in extreme sports such as bungee jumping and paragliding. Sport is a very good way to satisfy the brain's need for adrenaline. Popular and more accessible are non-team sports like running, cycling and boxing. The other direction is not so good and one which teachers need to keep a close eye on. Often, by early teens, boys in particular are looking for more risky and exciting activities. This can be smoking cigarettes, experimenting with cannabis or trying alcohol and before long can lead to them mixing with older boys who they perceive as more exciting than their own age group. These boys will often get them involved in petty crime and before you know it you've got a thirteen-year-old who is drinking, smoking and in trouble with the law.

SENSORY ISSUES

While more common with autistic spectrum disorder (ASD), ADHD children often have their fair share of sensory issues. These can be far-reaching. Some ADHD kids will have problems with food, for example having to have things served up in different bowls so food isn't touching, or only eating with their hands. Others will have issues with material they will wear. I remember vividly, as a teenager, hating anything that was nylon, wool or itchy. I've noticed a lot of ADHD people only wear cotton, jersey and denim.

Noise is another problem. A lot of ADHD people are extremely sensitive to loud noise, for example in restaurants. I've met ADHD people who don't like to be touched and others who have issues around certain smells. All the senses can be affected by ADHD and this is one that varies hugely person to person. There is no norm.

STEALING

There are a lot of ADHD traits that tap into this one. I certainly used to steal as a teenager and most clients I work with did as well. Luckily, for most of us, this tails off as we get near adulthood and realise that we don't fancy a criminal record. But … ADHD kids and young teenagers will almost certainly steal at some point. For most it starts with taking money from Mum's purse. The more serious will then progress to swiping Dad's credit card details or sneakily visiting the ATM with his debit card. Mostly this is the need for the adrenaline and excitement that stealing things brings. But there is also an element of our compulsive shopping and wanting bright, new and shiny things. Also, if an ADHD person wants something, they want it now! Right now! Saving up for things isn't exciting so they will very often take the money or steal the item because having it NOW is crucial.

SLEEP PROBLEMS

This can go one of two ways. Most ADHD people have trouble sleeping and this can start right from birth. Mums report ADHD babies needing little sleep and keeping them up all night. ADHD children often have trouble switching off at night, waking up during the night or waking up too early. On the whole, ADHD people need less sleep than others. Inattentive ADHD people, however, usually report the opposite. They can sleep like logs and many feel they sleep far too much. If you've a student who looks exhausted, has black rings under their eyes or who nods off in class, start asking questions. Do they struggle to sleep? Are they waking up a lot in the night? This could be an indicator of ADHD.

WANTING TO WIN/BE FIRST

Again, a lesser-known trait but one that applies pretty much across the board with ADHD. One of my clients told me that coming second was in effect losing and I have to agree with him. We do like to win and come first, which probably explains why so many top athletes and sports people are ADHD.

TOP TEACHING TIPS … Don't assume it's only hyperactivity/ distraction/inattention/impulsivity that constitutes a child's ADHD and the rest of their behaviour is them 'not behaving'. There are so many other ADHD traits.

WHAT WORKS BEST … Having a real understanding of ALL the traits that are going to crop up time after time in the classroom. And accepting that they are traits of ADHD and therefore considered 'normal' by the child with an ADHD brain.

Important stuff I want to remember:

TEACHERS! REALLY IMPORTANT STUFF THAT APPLIES TO ALL ADHD KIDS

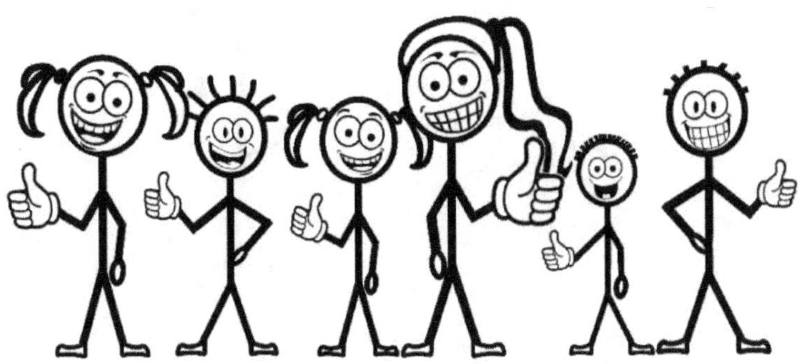

THEY'RE ALL DIFFERENT!

The first thing it's absolutely critical you know is that no two ADHD kids are the same. Never mind the fact that there are three diagnostic presentations of ADHD, within those you have hundreds of traits and dozens of comorbidities. Each ADHD person has their own concoction and the severity of all of them can vary dramatically as well. One example of mine: my inattention is severe but I rarely procrastinate.

So you might feel very confident that you've worked with an ADHD child before and can cope with whatever the next one throws at you, but you could be in for a big shock! Each one will be different. So saying to a mum, 'Well Jack is ADHD and he can sit still while yours is climbing all over the furniture,' is irrelevant. Never compare one ADHD child to another and never expect two to be the same!

I have been working with ADHD clients for ten years now, meeting thousands of children and teenagers all with the condition. I have yet to meet two who are even close to identical.

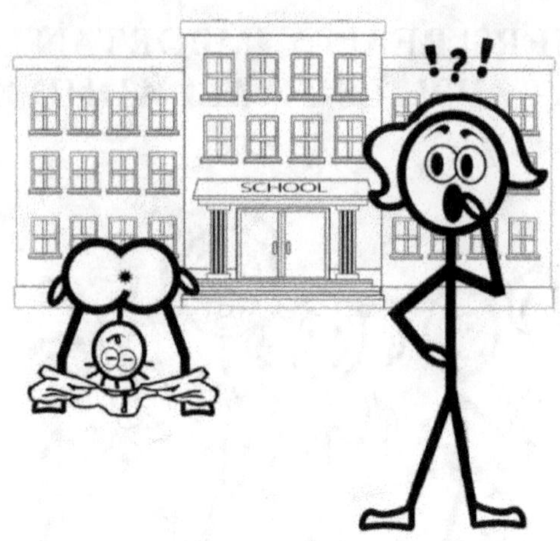

YOU CAN'T PUNISH DISABILITY …

Your immediate reaction to that statement is probably, 'Well of course you can't; that would be discrimination and we all know that's definitely not allowed. It's illegal, for goodness sake! There are laws about it.'

But have you thought that by giving detention to an ADHD kid who has been impulsively calling out answers without putting his hand up … or distracting others because he's bored … or rocking backwards and forwards on his chair because he can't sit still, THAT would be discrimination because ALL of those behaviours – i.e., IMPULSIVITY, DISTRACTION and HYPERACTIVITY – are traits of ADHD? And ADHD is a disability covered and protected by The Equality Act 2010.

But please don't panic that the next time you tell an ADHD kid off, you'll have the police knocking at your door later that night accusing you of discrimination. By the time you have read this book you will be so well versed in all the traits of ADHD that you won't be punishing any ADHD child for their natural ADHD brain activities, I promise you.

There are numerous other traits that we will go into in more detail about later in the book. But here's a flavour of some of the things that might be pushing your buttons in class but cannot be punished because they are caused by this disability:

- talking too much or interrupting

- forgetting to bring homework in

- being late for lessons

- not concentrating or focusing

- daydreaming

- fidgeting or swinging on chair

- doodling or fiddling

- calling out answers impulsively

And that's just for starters! More on this later though, I promise. And different ways of managing ADHD kids in the classroom means these issues should crop up a lot less over time.

Something that's critical to understand right from the start is that each ADHD child only has one brain. So every idea, thought, feeling and action comes from that one brain, meaning the question, 'Well is this connected to his ADHD or just him being naughty?' need never enter your head again! That's a defunct question. If the child has ADHD, ALL their behaviour is connected to their ADHD.

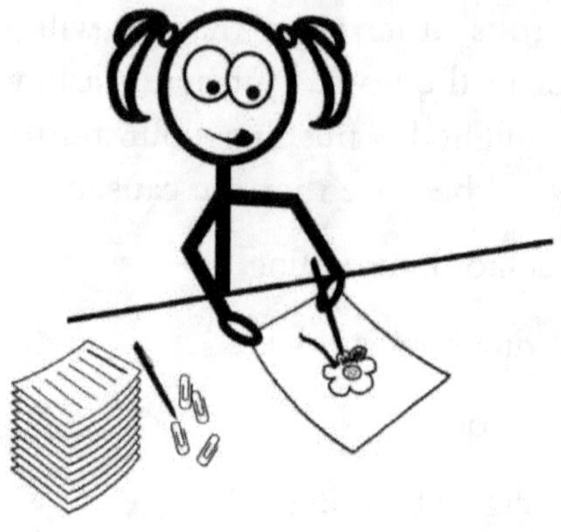

THEY'RE GOING TO BE INCONSISTENT

This can be infuriating for teachers, who are often understandably perplexed and can be heard at Parents' Evenings telling parents, 'I just cannot understand why she can concentrate, focus and produce good work in history and English but spends the whole of maths staring out of the window. She just needs to try harder.'

Err … no. Not if this is an ADHD kid. There will be something else going on and it's likely to be any or a combo of these:

1. This child has either undiagnosed ADHD and/or an undiagnosed comorbidity. In this case she could have dyscalculia. Undiagnosed comorbidities are so critical I'm going to go into them in a chapter all of their own. But undiagnosed comorbidities can explain why a child doesn't function well in one lesson but does in others.

2. She might not like her maths teacher. Simple as that. ADHD kids will respond well to teachers who treat them with respect and teach the subject well.

3. The subject where she's staring out of the window will be the one that is not stimulating her brain. If it's a subject that she is not interested in, and her brain does not find stimulating, you have almost no hope of dragging her attention away from that window and back to what you are trying to teach her.

These are the main reasons why ADHD kids are not usually 'good all-rounders'. They are likely to be brilliant at subjects they find interesting. They will probably perform best and try their very hardest when they like the teacher and the teacher treats them with respect. And they will be utterly rubbish at subjects that are being impacted by undiagnosed conditions like dyslexia, dyscalculia and dysgraphia. And they aren't going to give who they consider to be rude or unkind teachers the time of day, let alone make an attempt to learn their subject!

I can give you a very good personal example of this. Having come first out of 132 in maths at the end of my first year at my senior school, you might assume that I would have done reasonably well in my maths O level. However, I did not like my maths teacher. In my view (and that of others) she was rude, dismissive, constantly shouted rather than talked and was thoroughly objectionable. On top of that I spent four years not learning anything as I had already covered all this basic maths at my very good junior school.

So with a combination of these irritations, when I sat my maths O level I wrote my name and the date, then sat back in my chair, crossed my arms and thought to myself, 'F*ck you, you old witch. No; I'm not even going to do it!' I wrote nothing more and failed with an 'Ungraded'. It's not my proudest moment but it was definitely my undiagnosed ADHD!

Something which will help you with this is making sure that each SEND child in your class has an Individual Learning Plan (ILP) and is on your county's SEND register. They don't need an Education, Health and Care Plan for this, which is a common misconception.

If the child is at primary school it's ideal you get this in place ASAP. It will help each teacher or professional who comes into contact with the child be consistent and understand the child's needs.

If the child is at junior or senior school and no ILP is in place, it's not too late and you can initiate this as their teacher. On the ILP it will give you and their other teachers all the information you need about their strengths, challenges and any serious issues.

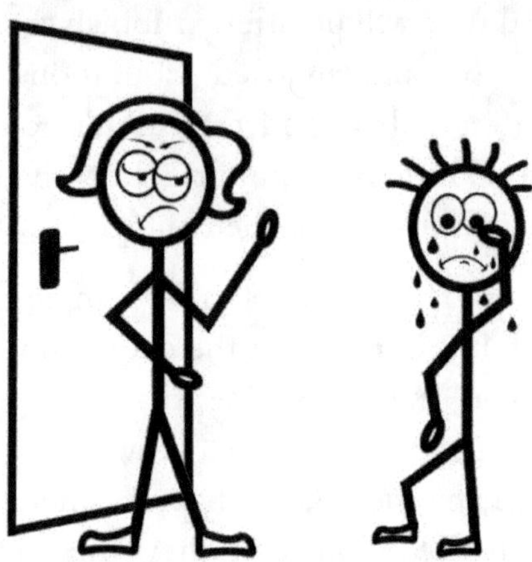

DON'T TAKE THEIR BREAKS AWAY

This is one of the first things teachers usually think of as a punishment. But it really is the very worst thing you can do to an ADHD child – both for them and, believe it or not, for you!

If your ADHD student has done something that genuinely warrants discipline, do your best to think of something other than removing their break time. Depriving them of their break does the polar opposite of what you want and will actually make their behaviour worse in the following lesson. There are lots of reasons for this, and I will go into more detail throughout the book, but just trust me; the last thing you want to do to an ADHD child is deprive them of their time outside, expending some of their excessive energy.

Important stuff I want to remember:

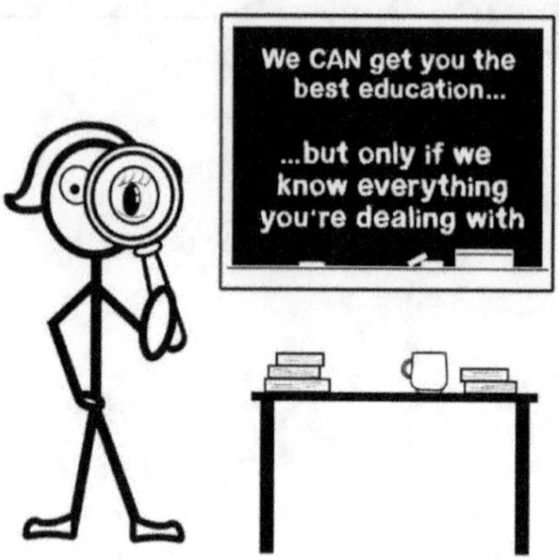

WHY ITS UP TO YOU TO SPOT THEIR COMORBIDITIES

'Hey? How did we get to the death bit' you might be thinking! Well we didn't – but we did get to what is otherwise known as 'coexisting conditions'. A much nicer phrase than comorbidities I always think.

So first up, a bit of interesting information for you. Did you know that 80% of people with ADHD also have one coexisting condition? And 50% of ADHD people have two or more. It's all to do with the brain wiring. And it means if you have ADHD you have a much higher risk of having any one of numerous coexisting conditions. And this is massively important for you: most of these are going to first show up in your classroom.

Having these coexisting conditions identified, diagnosed and (sometimes) medicated is going to be life-transforming for your student. Seriously, life-changing. So I'll go through the most common here to help you know what you're looking for.

DYSLEXIA

Particularly in girls, but boys too. This is the coexisting condition that DOES get picked up most – but still keep an eye out for kids who haven't had it identified. They will struggle with spelling, reading, sentence construction and punctuation, and may talk about, 'words jumping round the page'. They may reverse letters (e.g. 'd' for 'b') and muddle words that sound the same. Be very careful with dyslexia; I've yet to meet anyone with a dyslexia diagnosis who isn't also ADHD. However, once a child has the diagnosis of dyslexia their ADHD can be overlooked and all their issues assumed to be connected to their dyslexia diagnosis.

DYSCALCULIA

Sometimes called 'number dyslexia'. I have this one myself so can speak from experience. These kids aren't necessarily rubbish at maths, although some are. Others struggle with telling the time, get quarter-to and quarter-past on the clock mixed up in their head, jumble up long lists of numbers like mobile phone numbers and get different answers every time they add up a list of figures. We can sometimes be good at algebra or fractions but will struggle with other elements of maths. We aren't very good at getting tills to balance at the end of the day however hard we try and giving change can be a problem!

DYSPRAXIA

This is another one of mine so yet more personal experience! People with dyspraxia take clumsiness to another level. We fall over a lot, crash into doorways and furniture, struggle with doing up shoelaces, buttons and zips and often look dishevelled because it's very difficult to stay looking smart. We find it difficult to balance – as I found out when I tried a Segway for the first time. I was off that thing in seconds! No way could I balance on that.

We can be heavy-handed, breaking things when we don't mean to, press too hard on the paper so that what we're writing can be seen three sheets underneath and drop food down our tops pretty much every time we eat. We can often be seen in A&E, or at the very least with a myriad of colourful bruises from falling and bumping.

Something else to add here, which I didn't even know until my own diagnosis. Difficulties with processing can be a dyspraxic trait. I myself am diagnosed with 1% processing which, although it didn't come until my mid-fifties, made an awful lot of sense.

It's why I can never understand why anything works (like how to open packaging), why I can never follow the plot of a film and why I'm constantly pausing television shows to ask what is going on.

So if you have a child who is struggling to process as quickly as other children their age this could be linked to dyspraxia or, as it is now more commonly called, developmental coordination disorder or DCD.

DYSGRAPHIA

This is the least known of the big four Ds and in my view is the most crippling of all of them. In very simple terms, if you have dysgraphia the message your brain sends to your hands is corrupted. So while you might have all the answers and information in your head, putting that down on paper is almost impossible and offering a child with dysgraphia the use of a computer, laptop or iPad makes not a jot of difference.

SENSORY PROCESSING DISORDER (SPD)

This is a HUGE one and I reckon eight or nine out of every ten ADHD people have this. I do! It means we experience the senses differently. And that's all the senses, so it can affect smell, taste, sound, touch, textures, materials, food and a thousand other things. This will crop up a lot during the book as SPD plays quite a big part in a lot of ADHD kids' lives.

AUDITORY PROCESSING DISORDER

Nowhere near as common as its 'sensory sister' in my experience, but it is said between 3% and 5% of children have this condition. Very simply it means that the ears and the brain don't fully coordinate. So children might hear things differently, not be able to differentiate between certain words or sounds and process any verbal interaction more slowly.

OBSESSIVE–COMPULSIVE DISORDER (OCD)

In my experience not that many ADHD kids have this but the ones who do have it quite severely. My own view on this is it's because with ADHD comes overthinking and ruminating, which feeds into the OCD. OCD is when obsessive and compulsive behaviour has 'negative thoughts' attached to it. So for example a child might become obsessed around dirt/germs or checking behaviours, and if they don't do whatever it is, something dreadful will happen. I've seen ADHD kids badly affected by OCD, usually after puberty has kicked in. They need good ADHD-specific CBT for OCD. That really works.

ANXIETY AND DEPRESSION

These two conditions I can't stress enough. Both go hand-in-hand with ADHD. Either or both very often start around the beginning of puberty, which for some can be as young as nine years of age. The unlucky have both, but a lot have one or other more prominently. I was quite an anxious child but hid it so came across as a control freak and obnoxious. Boys will often cover it up with anger or violence. I'll go into more detail on this later in the book. But it's a serious issue for some ADHD kids.

EHLERS-DANLOS SYNDROME (EDS)

This is a lesser-known coexisting condition that can cause much pain at its worst. EDS makes the body tissue connections weaker. It shows up with kids being hyper mobile, so when one comes up to you proudly showing off how far they can bend their fingers back, they could actually be giving you a clue they have ADHD. EDS kids may have clicky joints, stretchy skin that bruises and breaks easily and wide scars that are slow to heal.

IRRITABLE BOWEL SYNDROME (IBS)

I've lost count of the parents who've sat in front of me telling me that their child has tummy problems, is gluten intolerant, lactose intolerant or being tested for everything under the sun when actually every single one of them has actually had IBS. Yet another one I'm diagnosed with. Mine came on in my late teens but I've known much younger children have this – even babies. So if an ADHD child needs to go to the toilet more regularly than other children, don't be surprised. And it's definitely worth flagging this up to the parents, if they haven't already noticed it at home, because there are some excellent anti-spasmodic tablets on the market that can hugely help kids with IBS.

ASD/ASC/AUTISM

It's generally estimated that 30% of kids with autism (or autistic spectrum disorder (ASD) / autistic spectrum condition (ASC), as some prefer to call it) also have ADHD. ASD is largely a condition affecting communication and social skills. It's a huge subject on its own but look out for socially awkward children, ones who find it hard to make friends, the loners, kids who struggle to integrate, the ones who aren't chatty and bubbly. They can be VERY bright academically and girls especially 'mask' well so it's difficult to spot, even for the professionals, so don't beat yourself up if you miss it.

TOURETTES AND TICS

Not a huge one this but I've had clients with both. Usually anxiety-driven and can be medicated. Also can be mistaken for impulsivity when kids shout out randomly in class. I've been guilty of getting this wrong myself, working with one lively six-year-old boy in therapy who was prone to shouting, 'FUCK OFF!' at the neighbours every morning on his way to school, mortifying his mother. I worked for weeks trying to control his 'impulsive outbursts' only for him to be diagnosed with Tourette's. I felt awful for not recognising it in him.

These are just the most common comorbidities and the ones that are most likely to crop up in your ADHD students. But there are others. Lots of others. Chronic fatigue syndrome and fibromyalgia are another two but these tend to come on later: mid- to late-teens is the earliest I've heard of. Alexithymia and dyslexithymia are another two: the first where people struggle to have feelings and emotions of any kind, even when they know they should do – for their partners or children for example – and the second where people struggle to name their emotions.

If you do start to see the signs of any of these coexisting conditions it's a good idea to keep notes of dates and examples. If it starts to build up into more than the odd example, that's when you need to have a word with your school special educational needs co-ordinator (SENCO). Bear in mind you might be asked to prepare a report in the future, especially if the child is going for a formal assessment, so it will help you to have notes from as soon as you started to notice anything that might indicate the child is struggling.

TOP TEACHING TIPS … Don't assume if a student has an ADHD diagnosis that's all they will be dealing with. It very rarely is.

WHAT WORKS BEST … If a child is struggling, ask their parents if they have been screened for any coexisting conditions. If none have been identified, keep your eyes and ears peeled for clues and dig deeper to find out what is going on.

You could be changing a life by picking something up in a student while they are still at school.

Don't think, 'It's not my place to do this; I am not a paediatrician'. Paediatricians don't diagnose comorbidities unless it's depression or anxiety. Nor do doctors. You really are best placed to spot the first signs of these in the classroom so please don't hold back! And involve the SENCO from as soon as you're aware.

Put reasonable adjustments in place while the child is under assessment, always collaborating with the child and their parents. They don't even need a diagnosis for you to accommodate their needs. Minor adjustments can make major differences.

Important stuff I want to remember:

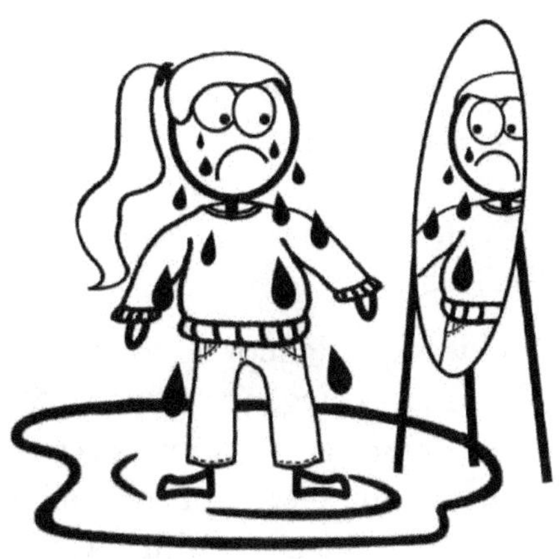

THEIR FRAGILE SELF-ESTEEM AND HOW TO HELP THEM HANG ONTO IT

This might be difficult to believe but an ADHD child, on average, receives 20,000 negative messages before they reach the age of twelve.

Just let that sink in for a minute. 20,000 negative messages before they even reach their teens.

Obviously this is an average and I doubt anybody's ever counted them exactly but it's very much the figure you hear used by ADHD professionals. Once you start looking at the traits it's not hard to understand why.

Speaking personally, during my childhood I was constantly and consistently told off for fidgeting, not sitting still, playing with and sucking my hair, not paying attention, talking when I shouldn't be, doing things too quickly, not concentrating on what I was doing, being very slapdash and clumsy, biting my nails, wanting everything my own way and being a control freak, mucking around and distracting others in class … I could go on.

In fact I will, just for a bit!

I was also told off for not looking where I was going, not letting people finish when they were speaking to me, doing things without thinking and without considering the consequences, taking over what others were doing, having no patience, eating too much, moaning I was bored, being hugely frustrated and irritated when I had to queue anywhere and being overly dramatic, oversensitive and a drama queen on very regular occasions. Oh and of course the big one: my ATTITUDE!

I'm perfectly sure I was quite annoying to others but what we have to remember is I was just being my natural ADHD self. Albeit with a hefty dollop of dyspraxia, sensory processing disorder and dyscalculia thrown in. But I can still remember some of those childhood comments now, in my late fifties. One of them was, 'Just concentrate on what you are doing.' Another one was, 'Why do you have to do everything in such a tearing hurry?'

Can you imagine how that feels? When you are, as far as you are concerned, doing everything absolutely normally and yet you get constant criticism for it. Well let me tell you, it wears you down. It makes you feel that you just aren't good enough, that by doing your best you are still annoying others. And that really can crush your self-esteem.

Some people are inattentive and blasé enough, like me, to think, 'Oh whatever; I will carry on doing things my own way,' but for some children this constant criticism can absolutely cripple their self-esteem and lead to feelings of self-loathing and most certainly feelings of low self-worth.

So let's think for a minute of the opposite. Let's think of a neurotypical child who doesn't do any of those things naturally.

Can you ever imagine saying to them, 'You're sitting far too still, you need to buck your ideas up, get moving and constantly fidget.' Or, 'You're being far too dull and boring today; can't you liven up and make yourself the clown of the class for a bit?' or, 'You're concentrating and focusing far too much. Show a bit of innovation for goodness sake and get your mind to wander off somewhere.'

Sounds absolutely ridiculous doesn't it? Nobody is ever going to say that. Yet we think it's perfectly acceptable to tell an ADHD child to stop doing the opposite when for them that IS their perfectly natural.

It's quite difficult to hang onto your self-esteem when you are a child, and particularly a teenager, with ADHD. What is natural for us irritates the pants off other people, especially if we aren't medicated. And a lot of us weren't and still aren't medicated because nobody has yet worked out we have ADHD.

So we've worked out that words are critical in helping your ADHD students stay positive and cling onto whatever self-esteem they arrived at school with.

There are always different ways to deliver messages positively rather than negatively and it only takes a bit of thought to come up with an alternative way of saying something that a child won't perceive as criticism. For example if they are fidgeting, 'For crying out loud can't you just sit still.' isn't going to be as well received as, 'Would you like to deliver one of these leaflets to all the classrooms for me. You'll do it quicker than anybody else.' Use their ADHD traits to make them feel good about themselves.

An ADHD child can't just magically make their ADHD traits disappear. Remember, this is not behaviour they are choosing. This is the way their brain is wired. So yes, ADHD kids will always try their very best to fit into the same pigeonhole all the neurotypical kids fit into BUT there are always going to be times when their ADHD will get the better of them.

I can't begin to tell you the huge difference how you word things will make. Be mindful of the language you use to try and get those 20,000 messages down to a more reasonable number! It honestly breaks my heart to think of five- and six-year-olds being battered by these 20,000 negative comments. Nobody would intentionally want to rain down constant criticism on little kids – but that's what happens when adults aren't aware enough of all these ADHD traits.

It's common knowledge that the self-harm and suicide rates are substantially higher for ADHD than any other neurodiverse condition or for neurotypical kids, so being really careful to word things in a positive way is going to play a large part in how the child feels about themselves.

Important stuff I want to remember:

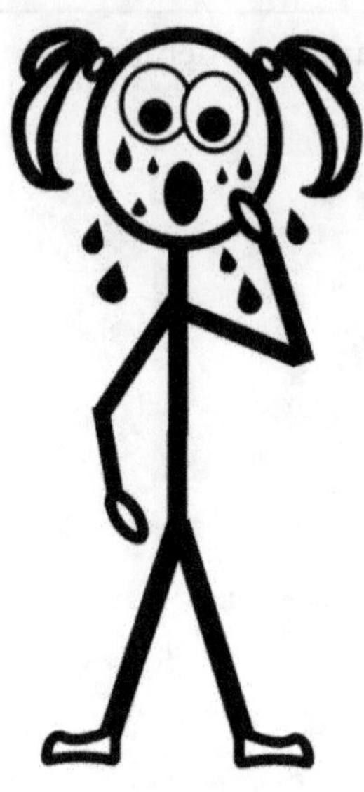

WHEN THEY GET OVERLY EMOTIONAL – EMOTIONAL DYSREGULATION AND REJECTION SENSITIVE DYSPHORIA

This is a biggie. It is now accepted in the medical world that the biggest impact of ADHD on a person is emotional dysregulation. Let's pause and digest that.

Not hyperactivity. Not inattention. Not impulsivity. Not distraction. Nope! Emotional dysregulation is what affects and impairs us ADHDs MOST.

For the scientists amongst you, google 'emotional dysregulation and ADHD'. There's lots of info online. But for those wanting the general gist, it means the bit of our brain that is supposed to regulate emotion doesn't work as it should.

I don't want to sound all doom and gloom but this can be the cause of serious mental health issues, so keep a close eye on the balanced (hopefully) mood of any ADHD students – especially teens when the hormone imbalance kicks in, too. Look out for this in girls particularly around menstruation time, as the combination of emotional dysregulation and raised hormone activity can send an ADHD girl into a whirling dervish of mixed emotions.

Not being able to regulate emotions can mean we become desperately upset when a TV character gets sick but don't shed a tear when a family member dies. The 'normal' emotional response often just isn't there. We either overdo it or underdo it. Our brain gives us no choice in the matter.

This can lead to some very inappropriate responses and an ADHD child may come over as unkind and uncaring. Actually, more likely they couldn't help wetting themselves laughing when the headteacher fell over and broke his glasses. You can see how this can get us into heaps of trouble.

The opposite can be true. You may find an ADHD student sobbing uncontrollably, awfully upset about something most people would brush off. This is when ADHD kids get accused of being overly sensitive or always wanting to be the centre of attention or of being a drama queen. Many a time, when leaving counselling sessions with young ADHD boys in prisons, I sat in my car and sobbed, totally overwhelmed and emotionally destroyed by their heart-breaking backgrounds and stories.

This is all standard stuff for a dysregulated brain. Add in to this something that is particular to ADHD brains alone: rejection sensitive dysphoria, or RSD for short.

There are two elements to RSD.

1. ADHD people do not take rejection well – and if you humiliate them, they will perceive that as rejection. So don't ever take the mickey out of an ADHD student! We might come over as bullish and strong willed and as if nothing would knock us down but it's absolutely not true. We are very sensitive souls inside and rejection massively hurts us.

2. The second element of RSD is ADHD people can perceive rejection when it is not even there. And we are SO good at this. If there's rejection to be felt, we will find it. And it will hurt. Just as much as proper actual rejection.

I can't stress enough how much emotional dysregulation impacts on the whole life of somebody with ADHD. It can be exhausting having emotions you can't control. Many a time I've been sitting down feeling perfectly happy when a wave of low mood has hit me for absolutely no reason. Only now do I know this is because of my emotional dysregulation. Half an hour later I feel fine and have no idea why I felt dreadful before. Before I learnt about emotional dysregulation, I'd sit wracking my brain as to why I was very sad or very happy.

I've had many parents tell me they can't understand how their child can be happy one moment and then miserable the next. They think the child is faking one or other of the moods. I can assure you this isn't the case. We literally can be happy, then sad, then happy, then sad, then happy, then sad – all in one day. It is genuine and it is exhausting to live with and there isn't a whole lot you can do about it apart from medication, which does even out emotions, when it's working properly.

If you have a child in your class who is often upset, make sure they have a safe place and ideally a safe person they can go to when their emotions are overwhelming them. You might think this will be more girls than boys, but actually in my experience just as many boys struggle with their emotions as girls, they just battle harder to cover theirs up.

TOP TEACHING TIPS … Don't chastise an ADHD child for acting like a drama queen for 'crying over nothing'. Remember their emotional response could be different to yours and everybody else's. Try not to accuse them of being overly sensitive or wanting to be the centre of attention because it probably isn't the case.

WHAT WORKS BEST … Allow your ADHD student to talk about how they are feeling. Listen to them without judging. Very soon their dysregulated brain will move them on from whatever high or low emotion they are feeling, and your best tactic is to not comment on them being moody or weepy but to listen calmly and wait for it to pass.

If possible, allocate one teacher, learning support assistant or member of staff to be each ADHD child's 'safe' person, someone they can go to in private if they feel overly emotional and need a non-judgmental, kind, listening ear.

Accept the fact that their emotions will be all over the place, especially during puberty, and try not to knee-jerk react to their mood swings. Remain constant; they won't be able to, but your kindness and consistency will help them regain their composure.

Be aware of the tone of your voice. Any sharp, harsh or critical-sounding comment will very probably cause RSD in your student and it will hurt them – however much of a cocky know-it-all they might seem.

Important stuff I want to remember:

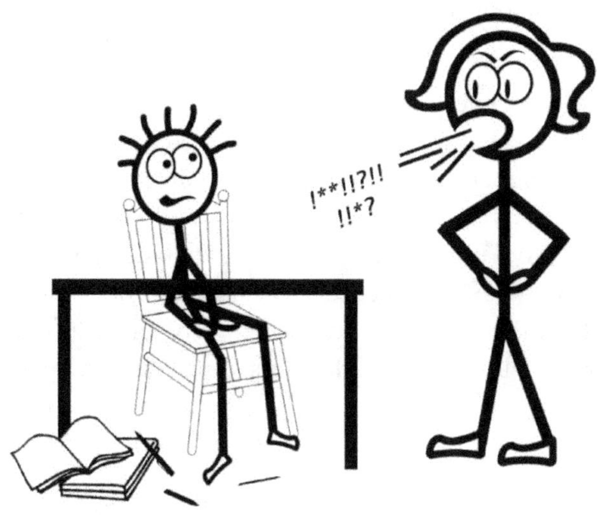

WHEN THEY START GETTING INTO TROUBLE WITH TEACHERS

It is going to happen. Even the best behaved 'got it under control' ADHD kids are going to hit problems at school for two simple reasons. WE DO NOT LIKE AUTHORITY and WE HATE BEING TOLD WHAT TO DO. These are consistent ADHD traits that apply to the Inattentives, Hyperactives and Combineds. So it is pretty much a given that schooling is going to become a problem. And as their teacher you're right in their firing line – with very little or, more likely, NO ADHD TRAINING. This is most definitely not your fault but it is shocking that teachers go through three-plus years of training and often don't hear mention of ADHD or ASD, yet you're then thrown in the deep end and expected to know how to educate and manage these neurodiverse brains, all with very different needs when it comes to learning.

As I write, in 2022, ADHD barely features in teacher training. I know, it is shocking! At best, you may be aware that ADHD is something to do with impulsivity, hyperactivity and distraction. And that usually is at best. I can almost guarantee you won't have been trained in the dozens of traits you'll be well versed in when you've slogged through this book. Hopefully as years go by this will improve but, of the many teachers I know, three hours in three years of training seems to be about the norm.

If you're lucky, problems won't arise until puberty hits from about age nine or ten onwards. ADHD is a hormone-connected condition so when those puberty hormones start jangling around their body, prepare to take cover. But a lot of ADHD kids don't run into major problems at school until their early teens. I didn't. Infant and junior school were pretty much a breeze, secondary school a very different story. But for others, from around the age of three upwards, not being able to sit still, general restlessness, distraction and inattention will bring problems from day one – even at nursery school for some.

For these characterful angels you need to start having regular communication with their parents. Don't assume the parents will know more about ADHD than you. Odds are they won't. Odds are also extremely high they have the same condition(s) as their child so they may think little Maisie is just fine, 'Because I'm exactly the same.' This is way more common than you think. I've met thousands of parents who think their child is perfectly normal having not realised they are severely ADHD themselves.

Because ADHD is a condition covered and protected by The Equality Act 2010 it means parents are permitted to ask for reasonable adjustments at school that take into account their child's disabilities. Each ADHD child will present differently and have different needs. For example, some ADHD kids need extra time in exams as they struggle to concentrate/focus on what's required and get distracted. Others need to be able to leave the exam early because they do everything at breakneck speed and will cause disturbance and disruption if they have to sit twiddling their fingers.

Reasonable adjustments you might want to suggest include a five- or ten-minute time-out card. This gives the fidgety, restless or angry child the time to nip outside for a run around to let off steam. Most schools will authorise this once a diagnosis is in place and, as that can be months, if not years, it should also be permitted while they're going through the diagnosis process. So it is worth checking school policy, and if it's okayed then offering it to parents if you see a child really struggling to sit still.

Fidget toys are a bit of a contentious issue. It is true that most ADHD kids need to fiddle, doodle, chew their pen, pen lid or pencil or do something with their hands all the time. It is the constant movement and stimulation that calms their brains down enough to concentrate. I know. Sounds weird. But it is true! If you want to see an agitated ADHD kid, ask them to sit perfectly still for five minutes.

I was a doodler at school and filled dozens of notepads with dot to dots, filling in the gaps or drawing random shapes and filling them in with biro pen just to keep me from going bonkers from boredom. I still do it today. However, it is also true that some fidget toys can be a tad noisy and a lot of schools have banned them for annoying other students. There are quieter versions, so raise this point with the school and ask them to agree to fidget toys that will keep the ADHD kids occupied while not annoying other students.

Wobble cushions are another option. They work beautifully for some, so worth exploring.

As ADHD kids gets older it is ATTITUDE that usually kicks in. Tons of ADHD traits feed into this. It'll almost definitely be a combo (or the full whammy) of having no respect for authority, not liking being told what to do, always thinking we know best, wanting things to be done our way and – the biggie – only respecting people who show us respect (not high on most teachers' list of priorities!) So from eleven-ish upwards things can go from being a bit rocky to 'off-the-scale nightmare' for ADHD kids at school. But if you know these insider tips on how to get the best out of their brain, I promise you it will be easier.

In my own case, from thirteen-ish onwards I simply thought most of my teachers were thick. Such was my arrogance! I used to point out their spelling mistakes on the blackboard with obvious glee. I was right, they were wrong. But I was 'mildly' badly behaved at school thanks to a strong-willed mother, who I was terrified of, sitting at home always ready to give me a rollicking.

Depending on the severity of the child's ADHD, coupled with the level of understanding and respect each teacher gives them, you could be in for some corker behaviour. Be prepared. It is not unusual for ADHD kids at school to throw things, kick things, shout out, talk too much, get distracted and struggle to concentrate. Their ADHD traits will be raging as the hormones do their best to unsettle them.

In nine out of ten cases, this is because they are bored OR think they are being treated unfairly. FAIRNESS is very important to ADHD kids. This is because we have that HEIGHTENED SENSE OF JUSTICE. So if something doesn't seem fair to us, watch out. You're going to get a reaction. And unlike a neurotypical brain, ours just won't let it go. Never in the history of a furious ADHD kid did the thought, 'Just let it go,' come into their outraged head.

So how can you help ADHD kids have a smoother journey through education? It is the C word. No, not that one. COMMUNICATION! TALK to the child and their parents. Together, explore and understand the idiosyncrasies of each child's ADHD brain. Be clear you understand what this particular child needs. Because ADHD presents so differently, as teachers you will never know exactly what each ADHD child needs. But the child and their parents should be able to communicate this to you. And be prepared for it to change as they get older.

It's a good idea to write up and keep some notes that get passed to each teacher the child is taught by. Give a trait that affects them, then bullet point underneath how this presents and how best to handle it. Something like this:

DISTRACTION

- He will look out of the window or be in his own head

- Ideally say his name to refocus him. Don't use Thomas: he prefers Tommy

- Shouting or humiliation will bring on anger

One of the biggest sources of problems is how teachers talk to ADHD kids. This is very easily rectified. What works beautifully for neurotypical children can press buttons in ADHD kids, but unless you've been told what these are, you wouldn't have a clue!

Shouting, raised voices, humiliating or talking to an ADHD child in a degrading way is a massive NO-NO. It's actually very simple. If you talk to an ADHD child with respect, you will get respect back.

The key is understanding that talking to an ADHD child in an angry, frustrated, irritated or demeaning way is never going to get the best response. I've been into numerous schools myself, training teachers, and almost without exception they gladly take on board that how you talk to an ADHD child is going to affect their behaviour and the performance you subsequently get out of them. Nobody has told them this before but without exception they have past experiences of talking to an ADHD child in a certain way which has always brought the best out of them. They have worked it out for themselves. Gold stars all round.

But there is always, ALWAYS one teacher who looks at me, steely-eyed, as if to say, 'Over my dead body.' And that is always the one that the child is going to come up against! Guaranteed.

Here's a very good example as to why it is SO critical to foster positive relationships between teachers and ADHD children.

I adored my English teacher. She treated me with respect and allowed me to read the part of Macbeth in class for two years solid for my O level. All the other parts changed weekly, but I suspect she'd sussed I was best kept occupied. So I enjoyed the classes, worked hard and achieved an A grade in English language.

My maths teacher, however, I THOUGHT was rude, dismissive, passively aggressive and in my eyes very disrespectful. Remember how I had outrightly refused to do my Maths O level because I loathed my maths teacher so much? There's not many who leave school with an A in English and a U (ungraded) in maths. But I did. And now I know I'm not alone.

WILDLY DIFFERING GRADES are an indicator of ADHD. Because we will work hardest in the subjects we love and where we respect the teacher. And our brains just won't get stimulated or involved in subjects we don't enjoy, or when we've clashed with a teacher.

Don't get the wrong impression. Nobody is asking you to grovel at the ADHD child's feet and accept disruptive behaviour. But an ADHD child is different and even in mainstream school reasonable adjustments are permitted for them to be treated differently, to put them on an even playing field with the rest of the class.

So do bear in mind that …

- shouting

- humiliating

- sarcasm

- singling out

… are pretty much guaranteed to bring out the worst in all ADHD children.

What works tons better is an understanding of ADHD and questioning rather than telling. I know many parents who have run reams of ADHD info off the internet, put it in files and handed all the relevant bits to teachers. It is well worth having a read of this if they do. Or jumping online yourself to find out more about ADHD and the particular subtype your student has.

Then to be mindful how you interact. It is always advisable to ask questions instead of telling. For example, 'How would it be if you tried doing that this way?' instead of, 'You've done that wrong. Do it this way.' The different ways those two different phrases are received by an ADHD brain are huge.

Questions work VERY well with ADHD. It makes us feel that we are in charge. Like our opinion matters. Like it is our choice.

Another issue impacting in class can be the ADHD trait of DIFFICULTY UNDERSTANDING INSTRUCTIONS AND DIRECTIONS. This is a big one in school. Our brains sometimes just don't know what the teacher means.

I remember very well the cold chill of fear that went down my back when we were instructed to pick up our pens and write when I didn't have a clue what I was supposed to be doing. A quick glance over my neighbour's shoulder usually sorted that out. Once I'd seen what the teacher MEANT, I could crack on and usually finish before anybody else. But struggling with instructions and directions is a much lesser-known ADHD trait and one you need to look out for in students.

Boredom in class is always going to be a problem for ADHD kids. Teachers are most often not aware what a major problem it is for an ADHD child to sit through even a thirty-minute class. Forty minutes is even harder and an hour a killer! It can be taking a monumental amount of effort to sit still, try to focus, not get distracted, not doodle and take in some of the information. You've no idea how hard an ADHD student is sometimes trying to do all this, against the odds, while the neurotypical kids sit there not having to try at all!

But the ADHD kids are so often going out of their minds with boredom. The answer? Keeping them busy and occupied. Being the 'clown of the class' is a massive indicator of ADHD. ADHD psychiatrists will always ask if this was you. It is born of boredom and not being stimulated and stretched enough. For example, I was an angel in English but a prize buffoon, always clowning around, in maths. Have a private chat with a child and see if any of this would help:

- moving about and being allowed to help you by collecting finished work, distributing handouts and other odd jobs

- running errands for you

- being allowed books to read when they have finished work early

- being allowed to do homework in class

Another ADHD trait possibly impacting at school is SOCIAL ANXIETY. Look out for this, especially in boys. It is one of the biggest comorbidities of ADHD. It could mean the child will be unexplainably uncomfortable (or downright bolshy) in groups, and this includes classrooms. They won't know it is social anxiety. And they'll probably cover up the anxiety by being aggressive and rude, even violent. I've worked with many ADHD offenders who can't even sit in a classroom at the age of twenty, because of the anxiety it causes them. This anxiety usually comes out in verbal or physical actions.

Something else critical to understand is that, in the vast majority of cases, no ADHD child is going to be equally good at every subject they are studying. While your neurotypicals might get straight A's or straight B's in all their subjects, it's much more typical for ADHD children to do extremely well in subjects they are interested in and appallingly when the subject doesn't stimulate their brain. Remember my A for English and Ungraded for maths! Not all will be as extreme as this but it's very unlikely an ADHD child will be equally stimulated by every subject they study.

This will hopefully allow you to be less perplexed as to why little Liam is doing so well in all his maths and science subjects and failing dismally at anything to do with English and creativity. It won't be a case of Liam not trying, and his school reports being filled with comments like, 'He could achieve in English if only he would focus, because he has proved he can in other subjects,' won't help his self-esteem. And with an ADHD brain this just isn't the case. They literally cannot stimulate their brain to learn or absorb information when the subject doesn't interest them.

I've worked with hundreds of clients where the children have felt tortured by being forced to study subjects they have absolutely no interest in. If possible, it's much better to let them drop the odd subject and focus on the ones they are good at. That's a reasonable adjustment that will pay dividends.

I was allowed to drop geography and science at thirteen and was very glad to see the back of both of them. Both bored me rigid. But in English, history and drama I flourished.

And when you are at the end of your tether with an ADHD kid, stop, take a breath and look at this group of people – all widely accepted to have had ADHD long before it was even as poorly understood as it is today! Can you imagine how easy it would have been for their teacher getting them to sit still, do as they're told and behave like other kids?

- Walt Disney
- Winston Churchill
- Stephen Hawking
- Agatha Christie
- Steve Jobs
- Joan Rivers
- Leonardo Da Vinci
- Elvis Presley
- Albert Einstein
- Vincent Van Gogh
- Mohammed Ali
- Wolfgang Amadeus Mozart
- Phineas T Barnum
- John Lennon

TOP TEACHING TIPS ... Don't expect all ADHD kids to be the same. They will all have different subtypes of ADHD with different severities, all have different traits and comorbidities and their needs will always vary hugely. Communication is key. Find out what they need.

They aren't going to be equally good at all subjects and this doesn't mean they aren't trying in the ones they are getting lower grades for. It could be linked to an undiagnosed comorbidity like dyslexia or dyscalculia. Or it could simply be that their brain has no interest in the subject and nothing you do or say is likely to change that, so don't waste your energy!

Speak to them with respect. You'll get respect back.

WHAT WORKS BEST ... ADHD kids can't help getting bored or distracted. Don't chastise them for it. Instead, work with them to find different ways of keeping them occupied and on task. But there will be blips. The way you handle them is the only thing that matters.

And did I mention 'talk to them with respect'?! You will be staggered at how much more they will respect you and want to learn in your class if you're not shouting at or humiliating them in front of their friends.

A good teacher who understands an ADHD child and supports them will lay the foundations for a very high-achieving adult.

So don't underestimate the impact of your input. It can be life-changing. My English teacher believed in me. My maths teacher gave me the impression she didn't give a toss.

Important stuff I want to remember:

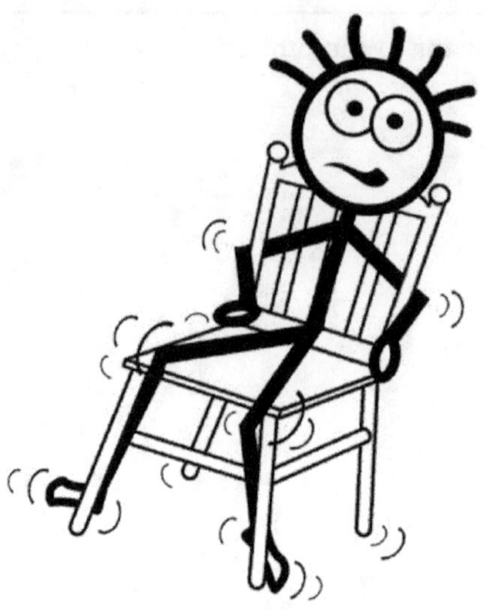

WHEN THEY WON'T STOP FIDGETING AND CAN'T SIT STILL

I'm guessing you've worked out the H in ADHD stands for HYPERACTIVITY … but have you linked that to the explanation as to why ADHD kids are constantly on the move? This is a proper problem, not to be taken lightly! We ADHDers have to keep something moving or we implode. I tried this experiment with a teenage ADHD client once. We challenged each other to sit perfectly still, arms flat on the armrest of the therapy room chairs, and we'd time how long we could sit. I don't think we made it past fifteen seconds. It was literally painful having to do it. Even we were shocked how little time we could sit still.

As a teen and as an adult I was constantly told to sit still, stop shuffling, stop moving and stop fidgeting – in cinemas and theatres particularly. The strange thing was I wasn't even aware that I was doing any of these things. But I must've been, because everybody and their dog told me I was annoying them by doing it. This was, of course, many years before my ADHD diagnosis. Now I understand that my urge to keep moving is stimulating my brain. And when I stop, my brain gets very frustrated and antsy.

So if your ADHD students are driving you nuts by tapping their fingers, fiddling with their hair, shaking a leg or keeping one part of their body constantly moving, now you know why!

My own way to occupy my brain in lessons was doodling. I would constantly draw big squares, chop them up into smaller squares and then start colouring them in. I must have coloured in thousands of squares over the years trying to keep my brain from dying of boredom. That, and swinging on my chair, rocking backwards and forwards. Until one fateful day I ended up flat on my back as the chair tipped over. That stopped me. But a good way of spotting ADHD in your class is looking for the chair swingers!

Medication helps with hyperactivity and restlessness a fair bit, as does having something in your hand to fiddle with. In every therapy session now I hold either a fidget toy or a pen and I'm constantly discreetly twirling it in my hand. If I didn't, I would get very anxious and wound up. It really does help to calm you down by having something to fiddle with. And by being calm, hey presto, we can think and concentrate on other things.

So rather than getting agitated with ADHD kids who can't sit still, understand that if they have the right thing to fiddle with that doesn't distract others, they are going to be able to settle and concentrate so much better. Find out what your school policy is on fidget toys, fidget spinners, wobble seats or anything that will keep their hands busy and body moving in some way. Ideally you want something that is not noisy and won't attract the attention of others but is stimulating enough to keep your ADHD student focused.

Also, take a lenient view when you are in the school canteen or somewhere else where the ADHD child is expected to sit for a long time. At lunchtime it's a much better idea to let them eat and then go off to do their homework if they want to, or go outside. Asking any ADHD child to sit at a table with nothing to do for a very long time is asking for trouble. Odds are they will be fine while they are eating, but straight after that they will be bored. They will need more stimulation.

To help with hyperactivity and restlessness, ADHD kids – boys in particular – need exercise every day. This really helps give the nervous energy an outlet. It also provides adrenaline, which calms their brains. So after lunch and at break times, if you can, get them on the field kicking a ball around; they're likely to be more able to learn in the next lesson and won't be so fidgety.

An absolute killer for ADHD kids and adults is queueing. We hate it and find it extremely difficult! Bear in mind that ADHD ID cards and Sunflower lanyards mean that ADHD kids (and ADHD adults) aren't expected to queue at airports, theme parks and many other places. So, whenever you can, keep an ADHD student out of a queue; it's almost impossible for them to stand around doing nothing. Give them a job to do instead, so they can keep moving. We don't have to queue anywhere else, so try to find a way to avoid that torture in school, too.

Team sports can cause problems – not always, but often. I've had many a teen client who has been sent off for accusing football or rugby referees of being 'totally blind' because they, the teen, know the rules better! Remember their trait of 'always knowing best'. They can't help it; it's how their brain works. And it's what will turn them into leaders and winners in the future. So listening to their point of view is always better than a straight, 'You're off, mate.' Adrenaline-loaded solo sports like running, cycling, swimming and climbing are usually safer. Boxing is also a great discipline and exercise option.

TOP TEACHING TIPS … Don't admonish them for fidgeting or not sitting still. Remember, they really cannot help it. Sitting still in classes for hours is about the toughest thing you can ask of an ADHD kid.

WHAT WORKS BEST … Make sure you have a ready supply of fidget spinners or fidget toys. Allow them to doodle. Understand they will be fidgety and will be shaking a leg or twiddling their hair. Allow them movement breaks. Use the ADHD kids to hand out worksheets or collect finished work from other students. Anything to get them up and moving.

Important stuff I want to remember:

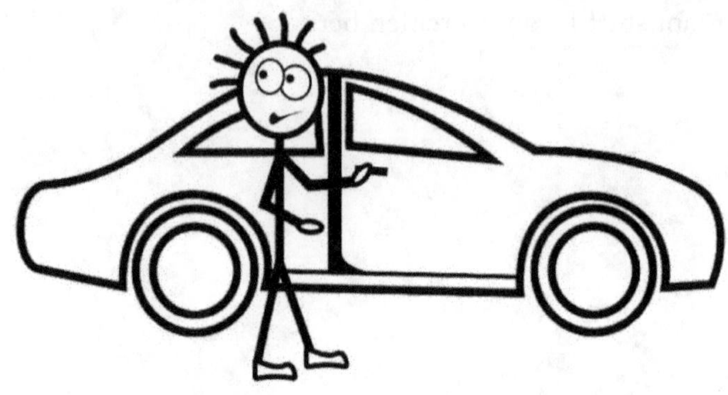

WHEN THEIR IMPULSIVITY SHOCKS YOU AND THEIR INABILITY TO THINK OF THE CONSEQUENCE DEFIES BELIEF

These are actually two separate ADHD traits but they are so closely interlinked they're going to share a chapter.

Impulsivity is when you say or do something without thinking. ADHD brains are incredibly impulsive – and the younger children are, the more impulsive they tend to be. That's not to say that teens and adults can't be impulsive, though, because they absolutely can.

Not thinking of the consequence is part of an ADHD brain's executive function – or should I say malfunction. Literally, the part of the brain that is supposed to think of the consequence doesn't work. And when I say it doesn't work, I mean really DOES NOT WORK. At all. No natural ability to think of the consequence of anything.

When you combine these two elements of ADHD, is it any wonder the prisons are chock-a-block with ADHD? As a rough estimate I would say 75% of the prison population is ADHD and it is their impulsivity and not being able to think of the consequence that has put most of them behind bars.

I have a perfect example. A young offender I was working with in HMP Portland was in prison AGAIN for stealing his thousandth car! I said to him, 'When you were just about to steal car number

1000, did it ever enter your head that it might not be a good idea? That the consequence might be you would end up back in here?'

His answer? When he had thought about it for a minute, he said, 'Honestly, no. I walked past a car, tried the door handle, it opened and the keys were in the ignition. What else was I supposed to do?'

He had impulsively opened the car door and the consequence of stealing that car genuinely hadn't entered his head – neither at that moment nor any time since – until I mentioned it. For anybody with a neurotypical brain this is really going to stretch your imagination. But I absolutely promise you it's perfectly true.

Our impulsivity and not being able to think of the consequence can be very extreme. A quick example of my own. A free newspaper plopped onto my doormat one day and on the back was a full-page advertisement for new apartments in Bulgaria. As I picked it up and made some excited squealing sound, my husband said, 'I don't even know why you're looking at that; you'll never buy one.' By the end of the day I had paid the deposit and was the proud owner of what turned out to be the most horrendous flat I've ever seen, in Sunny Beach, Bulgaria. An impulsive buy if ever there was one.

And the consequence was I lost a lot of money when I had to sell it for half the price and had never stayed in it once! The first visit with the estate agent was enough to put me off. But that hadn't entered my head as a possibility on the day I excitedly paid my deposit. The consequence of an impulse buy didn't enter my head until it was far too late and I was £25,000 poorer.

Adults with ADHD do impulsive things even when they are medicated. So spare a thought for children who haven't matured enough yet, haven't learnt to copy neurotypical ways; their little ADHD brains are going to be thinking and doing things impulsively all the time and they are never, ever going to be thinking of the consequence.

This is going to play out in numerous ways in the classroom. ADHD children will impulsively say all sorts of things both to other students and teachers. They literally open their mouths and the words pour out before they have given any thought to them and most certainly not thought of any consequences.

Especially when a child is not diagnosed, or diagnosed but not medicated, impulsivity and not thinking of the consequences are both going to feature on a regular basis.

ADHD kids will very often lose friends through this impulsivity; they will say something without thinking and cause great offence. This will hurt the ADHD child and they will feel bad about it, although actually they had no control over it.

If they are shouting out or saying things impulsively at school, understand that this is part of their condition. And that condition is a disability. So while you might be itching to send gobby Gavin to the headteacher's office, or even give him detention, for his latest witty quip that came out of his mouth impulsively, you need to hold fire and find other ways of managing it.

It's not unusual for an ADHD child to know the answer to a question and wildly flail their arm up in the air begging to be picked. When (in their opinion) they don't get noticed quickly enough, they can impulsively shout the answer out. If this happens in your class and that child is ADHD, diagnosed or not, then I promise you they have very little control over what comes out of their mouth. And because of their very poor short-term memory, sometimes the words will spill out because if they don't say it right now then they worry they will forget.

TOP TEACHING TIPS … Understand that the executive malfunction is responsible for your ADHD students' impulsivity and not being able to think of the consequence. This is part of their condition and needs to be recognised as such. The ADHD brain is hardwired to be impulsive and absolutely not think of any consequence.

WHAT WORKS BEST … Encourage the child to find ways of stopping and thinking before speaking. There are techniques and these tend to work better for older children rather than younger. I'm not particularly keen on it but one of them is that you put your hands behind your back and use your fingers to count to ten every time before you speak. Personally I wouldn't have the patience for it but it might work for some.

Be sensitive when pointing out to a child that they have said or done something impulsively or not thought through their actions and realised the consequences. Handled carefully, you can encourage them to be more aware of their impulsive actions and to try to consider consequences but do remember it is never going to be natural for an ADHD brain until it is medicated.

Important stuff I want to remember:

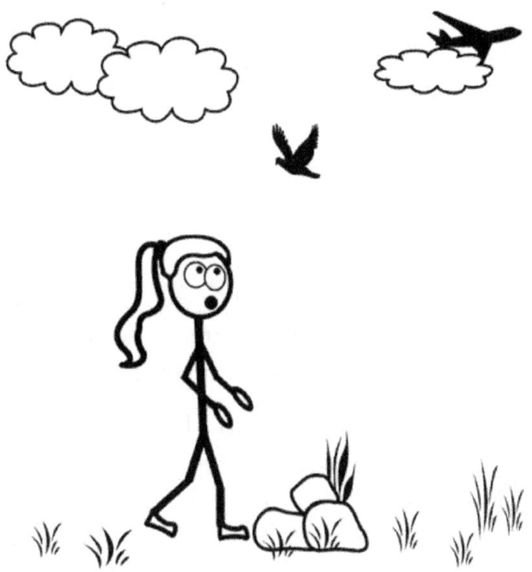

WHEN YOU CAN'T UNDERSTAND WHY THEY GET SO EASILY DISTRACTED

This is a nice easy one to get to grips with. Their ADHD brain is constantly looking for something more exciting. Easy to understand – but can still give you big headaches in class! If anyone is distracting others or being distracted themselves you can pretty much guarantee that is the ADHD kid!

You can also bet your life if there is something exciting going on like PE, drama or an activity where they are on the move, there will be a lot less distraction going on. But sit them down with an English exercise or a history essay and it's a different matter.

Distraction is a real issue for ADHD kids because their brain is always looking for something different. Something new. Something more exciting. Something to get their juices flowing. And this is a lifelong problem that you cannot cure just by being aware of it.

This is a bit of a random example, but I'll tell you how bad distraction can be. I have a strong memory of an English class when I was fourteen. I spent the whole fifty minutes looking out of the window, deciding whether I wanted to be an actress ON stage or do stage-managing BACK stage. I can vividly remember that whole thing in my head, but have absolutely no clue as to what was being taught in the English lesson! One thing I can be sure of though: it certainly wasn't enough to keep my brain occupied. And I LOVED English and my English teacher – but it still wasn't enough to keep me focused.

Distraction is worse for some ADHD kids than others. Some seem to be in a constantly distracted state and really struggle to focus and concentrate at all. For others it is a minor problem. But it will definitely rear its ugly head when anything boring crops up.

Always remember that this is their ADHD brain dragging them away from what it is finding boring to something that stimulates it more. An ADHD child's brain will choose for them what it focuses and concentrates on and what it gets distracted by. The child themself doesn't have much, if any, control over this.

ADHD medication helps with distraction. You should notice the difference if a student goes on it. Suddenly they will be able to focus and concentrate without too much difficulty, perhaps without ANY difficulty. It really can be quite staggering the difference ADHD medication can make.

There are ways of managing distraction. I don't particularly like any of them! Some children actually like to sit at the front of the class near the teacher so they aren't distracted by other students. Be careful about insisting on this, though, because there are those like me, where my anxiety was so bad that I had to sit in the back row of every class to make sure people weren't talking about me. Sitting at the front would've been torture. But if a child wants it (and some do), then allow them to sit as close to you as they possibly can.

For those who are distracted by what's going on outside the window – and a lot of ADHD kids are – putting them on the other side of the classroom might work. But expect an ADHD child to be distracted if there is anything going on outside the window, if there are any flickering lights or noisy or squeaky chairs, as pretty much anything can distract their brain.

Who they sit near is always going to play a major part in how distracted or distracting they are. If they are near somebody who is lively, possibly ADHD as well, they are going to find it much harder to concentrate and not be distracted by the other child. So careful placement of where an ADHD student sits is paramount when it comes to reducing distraction possibilities.

Also be mindful of overly busy walls. This can be terribly distracting for a child as can dangling anything from the ceiling above their head. Especially if it's moving: they won't be able to take their eyes off it. It's an idea to liaise with the child and, often, decluttering the area where they sit, so there are fewer distractions, works well in helping them to focus on the lesson.

How you bring a distracted child's attention back into the classroom is crucial and it's well worth discussing their preferences with them in advance. Clicking fingers or shouting their name isn't usually helpful. Most prefer something a little more subtle and less humiliating.

Back in the ancient 1970s, when I was at school, I remember teachers throwing blackboard rubbers at children who had become distracted. Or smacking a ruler down on the desk in front of the child. Thankfully we've moved on a bit from those days and often it's just a gentle nudge from their nearest classmate that's needed to bring them back from wherever their brain has wandered off to!

TOP TEACHING TIPS … Don't assume your ADHD students are purposefully allowing themselves to be distracted or telling them off for not concentrating and getting distracted, thinking they have a choice.

WHAT WORKS BEST … Understand why their mind wanders. Is there anything you can do about it? Talk to the child alone and ask them what would help. Each one will have different reasons for being distracted and may have thought of solutions themselves.

If they are on medication and still getting distracted a lot, it is worth speaking to their parents to see if they have had a medication review recently or are due to have one.

Always communicate to the parents that the child is struggling with distraction as this is something the parent needs to report back to their paediatrician.

Important stuff I want to remember:

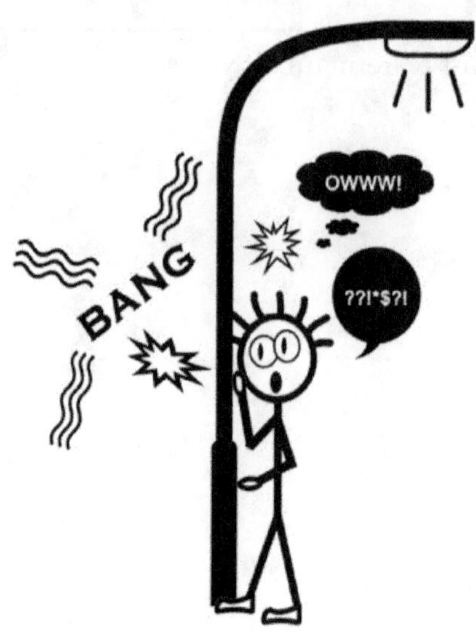

WHEN INATTENTION CAUSES PROBLEMS

The first time I realised how shockingly inattentive I was, was when I was doing the first of four driving speed awareness courses. (Yes, I know. Don't judge me. These courses are chock-a-block with ADHD people). We had to do a hazard-spotting test on the computer. I thought I was rocking it, clicking my little mouse every time I saw something hazardous on the road. I was sure at the end of it I would've spotted more hazards than anybody else. How wrong was I. I'd only spotted about half of them. This was years before I was diagnosed ADHD, so I just chastised myself for not looking hard enough. But it stuck with me. I didn't understand it.

The other time I shocked myself was in Tenerife. On the last day of a girly holiday one of my friends said, 'I'll meet you at the entrance to the swimming pool. The one with the snooker table.' I didn't have a clue what she was talking about. This was only a small hotel with two entrances to the swimming pool. And there were no snooker tables! Bear in mind this was the last day and I'd spent seven days going in and out of this swimming pool area.

After a five-minute stand-off with me insisting there were no snooker tables in the hotel, she walked me to one of the two entrances and – lo and behold – there was a big snooker table. I had walked past this thing for seven days and not noticed it. This was also years before my ADHD diagnosis, so again I just put it down to me being gormless.

Now I realise both these examples are because of my very strong Inattentive tendencies. From around the age of five I remember my mother wailing frequently, 'Watch what you're doing,' as something else went flying. I was forever knocking things over, bashing into things, going to pick something up and instead knocking it over. Neither of us knew why I did this, but I did it a LOT.

Now I'm older and wiser and know that inattention plays a very big part for most ADHD people. It simply means we don't notice things. And rectifying this is nowhere near as simple as you just telling ADHD children to pay attention. They can't. Their brain just does not do it. And trust me it's one of the hardest things to do when your brain isn't interested.

I remember trying SO HARD to pay attention in lessons and trying to force myself to listen to the teacher on numerous occasions. And again when I was at college, in my late forties, training to be a counsellor, the hours I spent trying to force my brain to pay attention when it was bored rigid and needed more stimulation.

So don't necessarily think a child isn't trying to pay attention because they could be making a huge effort to but still not managing it. Any of the following behaviour in your ADHD students could well be down to their inattention:

- falling over or tripping up

- knocking drinks over

- going to pick something up and missing it, so damaging or breaking or dropping it

- losing things because they've not paid attention to where they've put them

- not hearing instructions or directions because they weren't paying attention

- forgetting what they are doing halfway through whatever it is

- zoning out during classes – especially during anything prolonged, repetitive or lacking movement.

The list is endless. And while this is perplexing and infuriating for teachers, it can also be incredibly frustrating for the ADHD child. I so wish I could cure my inattentiveness, but it still features on an annoyingly regular basis.

Don't forget the first two words in ADHD stand for 'attention deficit'. That's how much of a problem inattention can be. Of the numerous traits it gets top billing!

So if a child tells you they didn't notice something or didn't see or hear something, and sounds like they mean it – give them the benefit of the doubt. If I can be incredulous about my own inattentiveness, then ADHD kids may well do things that stretch your imagination.

TOP TEACHING TIPS … Don't underestimate the impact of inattention on a child. And don't think that by just pointing it out to them, they will suddenly become attentive. It doesn't work like that! Don't ridicule them for not noticing things. That will just humiliate them, could bring on tears or anger and over time will definitely lower their self-esteem.

WHAT WORKS BEST … Look at different ways of doing things. If they are always knocking into a particular chair or desk, move it. If their attention wanders in class, agree with them collaboratively on how they would like to be brought back. Some just need to hear their name called out. For others that's humiliating and they'd prefer a gentle tap on their pencil case.

It's a very good idea to send any PowerPoint presentations you've used in class to the child and their parents. Not only will this help them with homework if they've lost attention during the class but it will also be massively helpful when it comes to revision. Turning PowerPoints into a slideshow is one of the best ways for an ADHD child to revise. It will be easier for them to hold attention and digest information as the slides move regularly.

And accept that there will be times when their inattentiveness will shock you. Try to see it as the disability it is rather than criticise it. Leave your, 'Are you as blind as a bat!' comments unsaid.

Important stuff I want to remember:

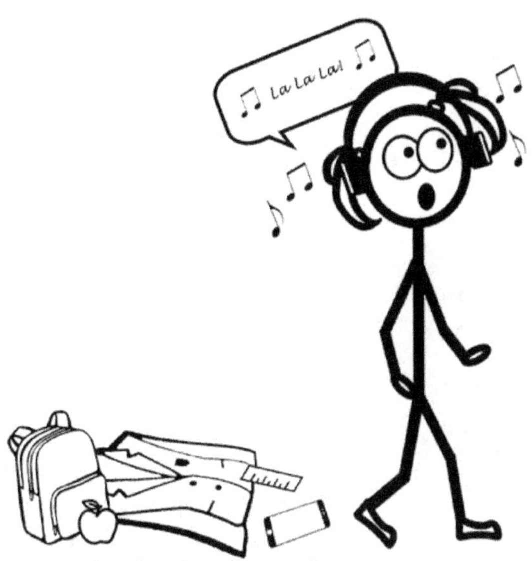

WHEN THEIR FORGETFULNESS IS DRIVING YOU POTTY

This is a big issue for anybody with ADHD. So a bit of scientific fact for you first. Short-term memory is a major problem for kids and adults with ADHD. Bizarrely long-term memory is usually fine so we can often remember things that happened five years ago but not five minutes ago. This is all to do with the brain wiring.

Don't forget what my first-ever ADHD psychiatrist told me: for a thought to become a memory it has to be thought for so many split seconds – and an ADHD brain rarely thinks a thought long enough for it to be stored as a memory. That really is a gem not many people know, even in the ADHD world!

So, first of all, get your head round the fact that an ADHD kid's short-term memory really can be shocking. It can be so bad that some young adults go to the GP convinced they have early-onset dementia because they cannot remember what they did an hour ago.

Your ADHD students won't be aware their short-term memory is poor, so sometimes they will outrightly lie and believe it is the truth because they genuinely won't remember. For example, your, 'Did you remember your homework?' question may get a yes answer because they've already forgotten they left it in the kitchen when they were having their breakfast and are quite convinced it is in their school bag.

It is usually when they start school that forgetfulness and short-term memory become a real problem, because it's the first time in their young lives they've had to remember stuff without the benefit of Mum's reminders.

I could list 100 things that a child can forget in a day, but common ones are forgetting to take their homework home, forgetting to bring their PE kit into school, forgetting to take the required textbooks in each day, forgetting to bring a school report or letter home, forgetting to bring their lunch, forgetting even to eat their lunch, forgetting what homework they need to do that night. The list goes on!

Before you read this book, you may well have become exasperated with their seeming lack of care and attention to these things but so much of it can be caused by almost zero short-term memory.

Medication does help with this and so do visual reminders. One thing you need to dispense with is attempting to get ADHD kids to remember to do things by keeping it in their head. That's a complete and utter waste of time. An ADHD child needs a visual reminder to remember to do things. This is when Post-it notes come in extremely handy. I have clients who have put Post-it notes in school lockers saying: 'Tuesday – don't forget to bring your homework/PE kit/lunchbox home'. This works.

So allow reminders on their phone if they're allowed to have their phone before/after school. Even if they have their phone back at the end of the school day, alarms set for each day, labelled with what they need to take home, will help so much.

And suggest to parents they have reminders in their bedroom to take things in to school on each day. These need to be highly visible. They need to be bright. And ideally they need to be movable, like a Post-it note, so the child can carry it with them as they move through the house as, trust me, an ADHD child can forget something when moving from one room to another. As can ADHD adults!

And anything that can be emailed to Mum or Dad that will act as a reminder, for example to do certain homework, is always a safer bet than expecting the child to remember.

Writing reminders in a notebook is no use at all because an ADHD child can easily forget to take the notebook or forget in which notebook they wrote things. Seriously. I do this all the time. I've given up with notebooks now because I only like new ones, use the first couple of pages, get bored and want a new one and then can't find the right one when I need whatever information it is I've written down!

This is why Post-it notes are so fabulous. They are cheap, colourful, bright and can be moved around with the child. They also give satisfaction and a self-esteem booster shot when the child screws them up and throws them away knowing that something has been achieved.

Short-term memory is worse for some people than others. Mine was fine as a child but worsened as an adult. Now it's appalling!

An ADHD child can also forget which class they are supposed to be in, what homework they are supposed to have done, what food they were supposed to have brought in for food tech lessons and literally hundreds of other things that come so naturally to people without an ADHD brain.

Be gentle with an ADHD child who says they have forgotten something. Chances are very high they will be beating themselves up for it before you even realised they had forgotten something. It's infuriating and frustrating for them so they need empathy and techniques for remembering next time rather than an exasperated sigh or a ticking off.

TOP TEACHING TIPS … Try your level best to be patient with a child who forgets to do lots of things. Don't roll your eyes heavenwards when they've forgotten something AGAIN. Don't ridicule them or humiliate them. They almost certainly can't help it and will often be as annoyed with themselves as you are.

WHAT WORKS BEST … Talk to the child about what they think might work for them. Make suggestions and try out new memory-jogger systems. Make it a fun learning experience with them as to what works to prod their memory and make their life easier – and what doesn't.

And if the school budget allows, put Post-it notes on a recurring order from Amazon! And if not, ask their parents if they can stick a pad in their school bag and use it frequently!

Important stuff I want to remember:

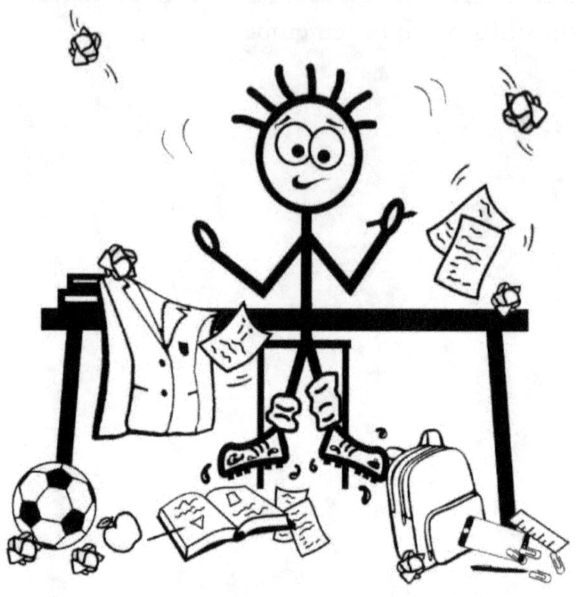

WHEN THEIR DISORGANISATION IS CAUSING CHAOS

Disorganisation and ADHD go hand-in-hand. What you need to remember is we have disorganised brains! So having disorganised schoolbags, desks, PE kits, pencil cases (and – at home – bedrooms, wardrobes and drawers) is the natural progression of that.

You might be one of the lucky ones, having a student who has at least a sprinkling (or as in my case, a large dollop) of perfectionism, which means they will have to have everything very neat and ordered. But this brings with it its own problems because these kids will have a right strop if anything of theirs is not the right way round, facing the front and in its place.

I remember being livid once a week, on the day the cleaner had been. She always moved my personal stuff and it incensed me. But the ratio of ADHD kids with perfectionism is small, so you are much more likely to be dealing with disorganised chaos in pretty much every area of their life.

Before we set about making the best of this, do spare a thought for their ADHD brains. Sometimes kids really want to be organised and they look at their neat and tidy friends in awe at the ease with which they maintain their orderliness. I used to. Much as I wanted my satchel and pencil case – and at secondary school my huge school bag – to be immaculate, it just didn't happen. No matter how many times I emptied it and put everything back in neatly, it always ended up in chaos. Within hours. This really perplexes ADHD children because they try harder than others to be tidy, but fail more. We just don't seem to have that neat and tidy gene.

You are never going to change an ADHD kid into that effortlessly organised child, but there things you can do to help.

Something important for you to know before we make plans is that they say with ADHD, 'If we can't see it, it doesn't exist.' This will mostly be obvious at home but will be useful for you to understand too.

If a child is walking round in the same pair of socks, the same T-shirt and the same shorts for weeks on end, this is because they were on the top of the pile! We will literally only grab what we can see because we don't have any memory of what else we own. If yours is a school where kids wear uniform, this trait won't trouble you much.

At my grand old age of fifty-something, I still wear the same five tops and four pairs of jeans on a regular basis. I have no time for the other 90% of my wardrobe, which I will only have a good root through if I'm going out for a special event. Because we do everything so quickly, and because we have no memory, we literally are going to wear the things that are visible. I'm constantly surprised by what I own when I have a good clear out. I have no memory of buying at least half of it and nearly all of it has never been worn.

So the answer to helping ADHD kids not be disorganised is largely by keeping 'stuff' to a minimum and their life as structured and organised as possible. This is not easy because other ADHD traits propel us into the complete opposite: our need for new things, our compulsive buying, our desire for the next thing or something different. We can so easily overwhelm ourselves and with overwhelm comes disorganisation and feeling, 'I can't cope. It's all too much.'

Disorganisation will often mean ADHD kids will turn up for an important football tournament having forgotten their football boots. Or to the opening night of the school play without their costume. Or to an English lesson without the text book that's lying on their bedroom floor.

Forcing organisation on an ADHD child is hard. Some will struggle much more than others with this trait. And, generalising, boys struggle more than girls – with some exceptions, of course.

So try your best to have the patience of a saint when the ADHD kid wails, 'I can't play football now,' and is blaming all and sundry for the forgotten boots. I can guarantee they are angry with themselves but it might not look like it. So be kind. Make it okay, some way – however you can. Beg, borrow or steal some boots or give the child the 'much more important job of refereeing', or ask them to, 'sit here with me to decide who should be in the school team – I need your advice.' SOMETHING to make them feel better.

And obviously don't ever penalise them for something they genuinely can't help and almost definitely annoys them more than it does you.

TOP TEACHING TIPS … Don't expect them to be as organised as other kids. It's very unlikely. And expect them to forget things. It's going to happen. Where you can, help them organise themselves and usually keeping things simple is the best policy.

WHAT WORKS BEST … Understand that being organised is usually frustratingly out of reach for even the most diligent and hard-working ADHD kids. They might want it desperately but, however hard they try, their disorganised brain will always win. So go easy on them and don't let them beat themselves up if they tend to get angry with themselves. Make it as okay for them as you possibly can. Have spare football boots!

And if there's anything very important they REALLY need to bring into school the next day, like the school play costume, always message their parents.

Important stuff I want to remember:

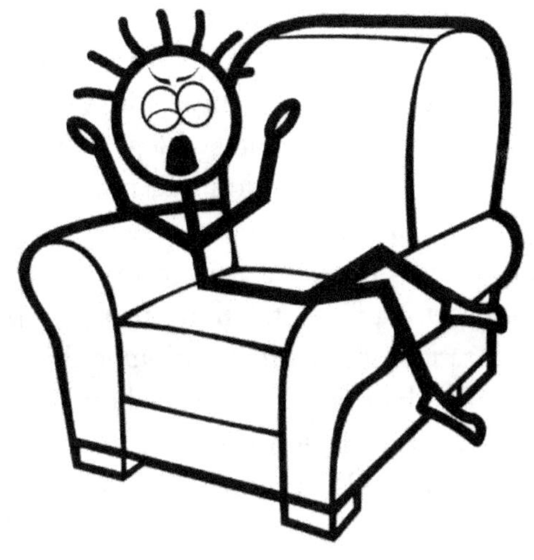

WHEN THEIR PROCRASTINATION IS WINDING YOU UP

Now this trait is a lot stronger for some with ADHD than others. Personally, I rarely have it unless something is exceptionally boring, like accounts! Mostly, people with Hyperactive or Combined ADHD don't procrastinate anywhere near as much as people with Inattentive ADHD. However, we ALL become masters at it when something is extremely boring. But it is those with Inattentive ADHD who seem to be able to procrastinate over just about everything and this can be perplexing and frustrating for them as well as infuriating for those around them.

What we have to remember with ADHD kids is procrastination IS an ADHD trait. They are not just being slow coaches or lazy layabouts to purposefully get on your nerves or because they can't be bothered. What their brain is actually saying to them is, "this isn't exciting enough for me to get stimulated about so I'm not doing it. At most I might do it later. But the odds aren't good."

Lack of motivation and procrastination are right high up there in the list of how ADHD 'impairs' somebody. Sometimes our procrastination even drives US nuts but there is very little we can do about it.

Yet again it is medication that can make the world of difference. A little example for you on that. One morning when I took a stimulant medication, I spent two and a half hours sorting out some receipts and accounts that I had been ignoring avidly for the past year. It wasn't until that afternoon that it suddenly clicked why I had managed to do it: the procrastination had been eradicated by the medication. So if parents have been putting off medicating their diagnosed child, or even pursuing a diagnosis for an undiagnosed child, and you are seeing procrastination as a major problem that's affecting their education, it's worth mentioning this to the parents. Obviously you can't TELL a parent to medicate their child, or to seek a diagnosis, but you can inform them that procrastination is now causing a problem and you know it's one of the traits ADHD medication can help.

There are a few tried-and-tested ways round procrastination, but before we move onto those, I must let you know of another reason why ADHD people sometimes procrastinate. Believe it or not it's perfectionism. Perfectionism can be part of ADHD and it can make a lot of kids and adults procrastinate. Their thinking is that unless they can do something perfectly, they don't want to do it at all.

I've met grown ADHD adults who have procrastinated for years because they weren't sure they could do a complete project properly. So what could look like chronic procrastination to you, might actually be an ADHD child wrestling with a project, thinking if they can't do it perfectly what's the point of doing it at all. And they will always need a reason why. More on that in an upcoming chapter but for now just trust me, they will do!

The best way to motivate an ADHD child to do something, if they are procrastinating, is to give them a reason to do it. That reason usually needs to be in the shape of a reward. I remember as a child only being motivated to do my homework if I did it BEFORE my tea. If I'd left it till AFTER tea there was just no reason to do it, nothing to look forward to! I had to have the reward of dinner to look forward to in order to get through the homework. Unknowingly, I had worked out how to handle my ADHD from quite a young age. I'm talking around eight or nine years old.

This is actually quite a simple trait to handle. Whatever it is you want the child to do, try to make sure there is something nice at the end of it. It doesn't have to be something costly. For me it was just my dinner every night that made me do my homework. For ADHD kids in your class it could be encouraging them to finish something before break or lunchtime – and the promise of an extra ten minutes on the playing field if they get a piece of work finished.

Admittedly, it is easier to put rewards in place at home and I totally appreciate resources are limited at school so you will need to think creatively and obviously take their classmates into account! You can't be seen to be favouring the ADHD child but you can be seen to do things differently if it motivates them.

At home they might get access to their iPad when they have finished their homework. A lot of parents of ADHD children I know say that there is no television until homework is done. You need to stick to similar rules at school because they do work. Nothing motivates an ADHD child like a nice big juicy carrot at the end of something boring.

ADHD kids will find plenty of things to procrastinate over, not just their school work, but the same rules always apply. They will need a reason to do something and that can be a very simple reward like leaving the classroom two minutes early so they can be first in the lunch queue, or being put in charge of choosing who plays for which netball team. Their brain needs something to aim for and a reason to do something.

And if perfectionism is the problem, encourage the child to do a small amount of whatever it is you are wanting them to conquer. Let's say it is a craft project that they just can't get started on, for no reason you can think of. Encourage them to start with just one small area. Maybe think about what colours they want to use or what materials.

And if it's an essay they are struggling to get started on, suggest they start in the middle with the main content and write the introduction afterwards. This works for a lot of kids who struggle to get started. Or maybe they could bullet point ideas and then turn those into an essay. Allow them to see that they can do small chunks perfectly and then move onto the next section.

ADHD overwhelm means that sometimes we can procrastinate because a task becomes overwhelming and we don't think we can do it perfectly. So breaking things down into much smaller chunks often works.

Goal-setting also helps with ADHD procrastination. If an ADHD child is procrastinating over a lot of things, odds are they are struggling with overwhelm at the same time. Writing things down, either in a diary, journal, notebook or on their phone (when allowed) can make things look a lot less overwhelming. Get it out of their head so they stop overthinking it. Written down, things always look much less overwhelming to an ADHD child. And subsequently they procrastinate less. Just don't expect them to ever be able to find that notebook again!

Think about helping the child to schedule getting tasks done, and focusing on how they will feel at the end of it. ADHD people tend to get overwhelmed and despondent when they look at the bigger picture.

Encourage the child to look at the small picture. If they complete one tiny project/paragraph/piece of work every day, at the end of the week they will have achieved five things – and at the end of the month, twenty! I guarantee you they will never have thought of it like that.

You can motivate an ADHD child by explaining if they just spend however many minutes each day, by the end of the month they will have chalked up twenty achievements. And the cherry on top will be if you give them a reward for achieving five things AND also for twenty things.

TOP TEACHING TIPS … Don't show them up by pointing out how everybody else is getting on with a task, why they need to just get cracking, get on with things, and to stop making excuses. Procrastination is part of their brain wiring and not so easily overcome.

WHAT WORKS BEST … Talk to them about what needs doing. Try to understand their thoughts on the issue. Ask them what would motivate them to achieve whatever needs doing. Do they understand what is being asked of them?

Make sure they feel in charge of how they go about things. Help them make a schedule and set goals to achieve tasks. Set them rewards for achieving whatever needs to get done.

Important stuff I want to remember:

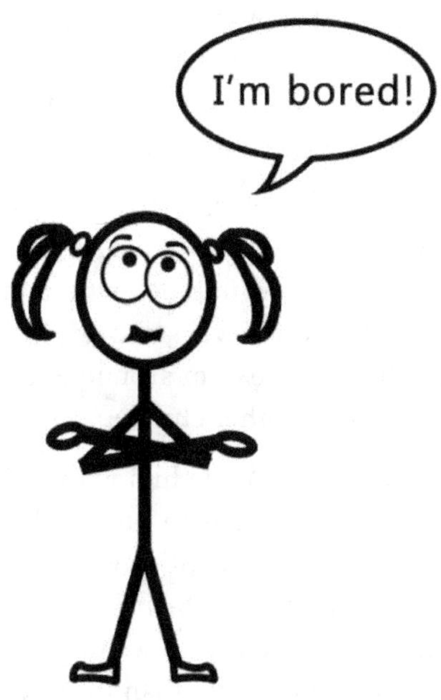

WHEN THEY'RE CONSTANTLY MOANING 'I'M BORED'

Whichever sort of ADHD you're dealing with in your class I can pretty much guarantee you are going to hear this often: 'I'm SOOOOO bored!'

Firstly, don't chastise them for it. An ADHD brain needs a lot of stimulation and the minute it doesn't get it, yes, it IS bored. When you hear a child say they are bored, replace the B word in your brain with 'under-stimulated', because that's what they mean. They just don't understand that yet.

I remember being told the word 'bored' was banned when I was young because I used it so often. And I was always being told to go and read a book. Which was fine, and I did, until I became bored with that, too.

This is a very easy trait to understand. An ADHD child's brain needs and craves more stimulation than a normal brain. It is constantly looking for excitement, for something new, for something different and for something challenging. The right medication helps hugely with this and should allow the child's need for 'something more' to calm down. An unmedicated ADHD child, however, will be forever searching for something new and exciting to do. And if it can't find it, this is the point when you will hear the wail of, 'I'm BORED.'

There are lots of things that help with this. Daily exercise is a brilliant way for any ADHD child to receive the right dose of adrenaline. Unless it is tipping with rain, get the ADHD child outdoors and active. Never take away their break time as a punishment; they need to run around and release all their pent-up energy more than any other children.

In class it's often the ADHD child who will finish their work first. Their brains work quicker than others. And that's when boredom will kick in. There are loads of ways you can manage this though; and trust me you do need to 'manage it' because there's little hope of them just sitting quietly and waiting for others to finish! Their brain needs more stimulation than that. So if you don't want them risking breaking their neck by rocking backwards and forwards on their chair, chatting to and distracting their mates or idly picking holes in their school jumper, keep them busy.

Ideas that work are allowing them to do their homework once they've finished their work. Or allowing them to read a book. Or asking them to hand out worksheets, marked homework or anything else that needs plonking on classmates' desks.

And if you need errands running, you'll find the ADHD kid more keen than most to whizz off to another classroom or to take something to the headteacher.

If you're a teacher with ADHD kids of your own, always have a ready supply of whatever it is that excites your child's brain at home. If it is arts and crafts, always have a good supply and introduce new bits every time. It doesn't matter how cheap and cheerful they are, because anything new will count as exciting to an ADHD child when they're young. It can be literally a different piece of coloured cardboard or a pack of cheap felt pens. An ADHD brain is easily fooled when they're little: if it is new, it is exciting. As they get older 'exciting' becomes a bit more expensive and is usually in the shape of trainers or devices.

At home try to break up activities, especially during school holidays. It is not good to leave an ADHD child with absolutely nothing to do all day. Make sure there is something scheduled at some point of the day, whether that's a dog walk, a picnic, a swim, a game of rounders or a cinema visit. Whatever it is, try to add at least one event into each day, so your ADHD child has something to look forward to and get excited about.

At school this is tougher but any chance you have to get them out of the classroom, onto the field or into the gym, music room, drama studio or art room, you are going to find the ADHD child is much more engaged.

Always be prepared for the post-activity crash. And this is the same at school as at home. It is always very disappointing for an ADHD brain when an activity ends, so make sure when you finish a PE or art and craft class where the child has been active, that there is something nice to look forward to. At home it can be as simple as a bar of chocolate; just give your child something to be excited by when an activity ends.

At school it's harder but keeping the child engaged is important. So if it's an English class they're going into, ask them to read the lead character in whatever Shakespeare they're studying. You need to keep their brain interested and stimulated. If you don't, the drop in adrenaline will make them at best surly and uninterested, at worst mouthy, belligerent and hugely distracting to others.

I can remember feeling very frustrated, unsettled and restless when I had to go back to doing something academic after a fun class. It was also much more difficult to focus and concentrate and made studying so much harder if my brain was flat after doing an active class like drama.

I've known clients to be absolutely bewildered by their child's meltdown when they come home from having had a lovely time out. The equivalent at school is coming in from a two-hour football match or a netball tournament. I know from my own experience, even now, this is because of the sudden drop in activity levels. Once that adrenaline stops pumping, any ADHD child is going to get very grumpy if there is nothing nice to look forward to.

ADHD kids can get bored with anything and that includes people. So if you see an ADHD kid joining and leaving friendship groups on a regular basis it's not necessarily anything to worry about; they may well just be bored with that group's activities or conversation and fancy a change!

Above all, ADHD kids need to be kept occupied. For those without social anxiety, sign them up to as many clubs as they are interested in. Encourage them to join any lunchtime and after-school clubs or groups. Sports, drama, dance or singing are all good choices. Encourage them to be active as much as you possibly can.

And when it's appropriate, give them responsibility. Whatever chores need doing in your classroom or on the sports field, ask the ADHD child if they would like to do it first, and give them a nice flash title to go with it. Trust me, the boredom levels will lower instantly.

TOP TEACHING TIPS … Don't tell them it is wrong or irritating or too demanding to keep saying they're bored. Don't insist they CAN'T be bored with a two-hour essay still needing to be written. If their brain isn't stimulated by whatever you are asking them to do, their natural reaction is going to be to declare, 'I'm bored.' Remember, this is their only way of communicating to you that their brain is under-stimulated.

WHAT WORKS BEST … Understand that this is just how their adrenaline-seeking brain works. They can't help it.

Communicate and collaborate with them about what it is they want and need to do to stop feeling bored. Encourage daily creative and sporting activities, lunchtime and after-school clubs.

If you're also the parent of an ADHD child, become a frequent visitor to Poundland or other cheap shops, picking up colourful and interesting little bits in the arts and craft, and the stationery sections.

Pre-empt the post-activity crash by having something nice or stimulating lined up for afterwards.

Important stuff I want to remember:

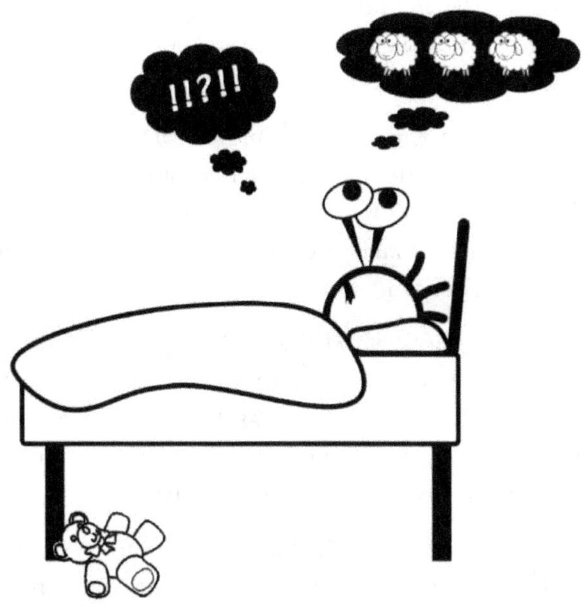

SLEEP PROBLEMS AND HOW THEY IMPACT AT SCHOOL

Sleep is a big problem with ADHD. In fact, it is only very recently they've decided that having a sleep disorder isn't a comorbidity of ADHD: it is part of the condition.

Parents of ADHD kids are likely to hit problems with sleep early on, and often report babies who never slept or took hours to settle or needed constant stimulation. These babies grow into Hyperactive or Combined ADHD toddlers. On the opposite end of the scale, generally Inattentive babies are sleepy-heads who will sleep forever. And they get very grumpy when they're woken up.

First off, going to bed and sleep is BORING for so many ADHD kids who will fight the whole routine. They won't want their night-time shower or bath, to brush their teeth or get into bed because their brains are saying, 'This isn't exciting. Let's stay up longer and have FUN.' Yep, really! My brain still does this today. No matter how shattered I am, sometimes my brain just won't calm down and stop thinking.

So when an ADHD child starts kicking off about going to bed it is because their brain wants them to stay awake. Not just them being contrary!

For those of you with ADHD children of your own, and those of you working in residential units where you are putting ADHD kids to bed, I'm going to give you lots of advice and a good few ideas that help, but first of all let's deal with how sleep can affect an ADHD child in the classroom.

If you are noticing they're tired and sleepy, it's well worth pointing this out to the parents. They may well be thinking their child is turning the light off at 9 p.m. as instructed when in actual fact they're staying up till 4 a.m. on their Xbox. Another real life example from a strong-willed teenage client!

An ADHD child may have had a very bad night's sleep. Sometimes it can take them hours to get to sleep and they are very grouchy when they are woken up. This can make them tired and short-tempered in the class.

There are different ways of dealing with this at home and I always advise parents or carers the best way is to make bedtime more interesting. I hesitate to use the word 'fun' because what they are needing to do is calm the child's brain down. BUT there are ways to stimulate an ADHD child's brain enough to get it to want to go to bed without a fight.

So let's deal with getting an ADHD child actually INTO bed before we deal with getting them to sleep, which is a whole other ball game.

To get a child faintly interested in the bedtime process, I strongly recommend putting a reward system in place. These need to be highly individualised because what will float one ADHD kid's bedtime brain won't float another.

But reward systems generally work VERY well at bedtime. Because, quite honestly, going to bed and shutting down our brain is pretty much the toughest thing we have to do each day. And the torture is worse because it is EVERY DAY. Day in, day out! I know many ADHD adults who still hate the bedtime routine and find going to sleep the hardest thing they do every day.

So whether it's milk and cookies, or a hot chocolate, or an hour of reading time, try to find something that will motivate the child into wanting to get into their bedroom.

Let's assume we've got the little angel in bed with whatever reward system worked. (One always will; it can just be trial and error finding it.) Parents or carers now have the issue of getting them to sleep.

First of all, please never make the mistake of thinking it is easy! The 'just shut your eyes and go to sleep' routine will not work with most ADHD brains. I remember being told this numerous times as a child and it made no sense to me at all. Instead, there are tons of things you can do to help an ADHD child sleep. In no particular order they are as follows:

- Melatonin is recommended for ADHD children who struggle to sleep. Parents should be able to get this from their GP and it is relatively easy to order online as well. They can even buy it in a Gummy Bear from Amazon. Melatonin helps most ADHD children sleep and a lot of parents swear by it.

- Weighted blankets. I've no idea actually why, but almost certainly because of our sensory issues, a lot of ADHD children and adults like to have pressure on top of them; it makes them feel safe and protected and therefore more able to relax and go to sleep. Be careful because there are a lot of cowboys out there charging small fortunes for weighted blankets. There is no need to pay those crazy prices. Instead, look for a local seamstress who can make one or do a very thorough internet search before committing.

- Anything that will calm down an ADHD brain is always going to be helpful. Aromatherapy can be good. Diffusing some particularly relaxing oils, like lavender and chamomile, in the room can definitely help.

- Sleep hypnotherapy also works. Ideally, this needs to be played on a constant loop at a low volume: just high enough to be heard but not loud enough to be annoying.

- There are also some very relaxing projector visuals like moons and stars that you can play on the child's ceiling. Amazon is a good source for these.

- Reading is a great way to calm down an ADHD child's brain before bedtime. But make it a book or comics, ideally, not a Kindle. And always get the child off any screens a minimum of an hour before trying to get them to sleep, ideally longer. Do make sure any tablets or phones they are using switch to blue light rather than bright light from early evening onwards.

There are no magic answers when it comes to sleep. Insomnia really is part and parcel of having ADHD. And it is much more of a problem for some than others. For me it has always been the worst part of having the condition.

ADHD medication can also make matters worse. Parents need to be very careful if a child is starting on stimulant medication and it majorly impacts their sleep. They should keep in regular touch with their paediatrician, psychiatrist or meds prescriber because poor sleep over a long period can be seriously detrimental to a child's health. It can impact their mood, behaviour and performance at school.

Lack of sleep can also be dangerous because it makes kids distractible and far less attentive when doing things like crossing the road. Sleep is imperative for mental and physical health, but can be very, very difficult to achieve. It is really a question of trial and error, and trial again.

Something to be aware of is delayed sleep phase syndrome (DSPS). This is a condition not solely applicable to ADHD, but a lot of ADHD people have it. I do. It is where your circadian rhythm is approximately four hours out of sync with 'normal'. So instead of getting sleepy around 10–11 p.m., a DSPS brain will keep going until around 4 a.m. and prefer to sleep until lunchtime.

Not all, but most Inattentive ADHD kids have no problem sleeping. My Inattentive brother would amaze us by sleeping for whole weekends in his teens. Their problem is usually that they feel sleepy and tired too much.

But most ADHD kids have problems getting their brains to shut off, so I suggest parents and carers try everything they possibly can. My bedroom at night has aromatherapy, hypnotherapy AND prescribed sleep medication ALL battling to get my brain to sleep.

TOP TEACHING TIPS … Don't assume a child not sleeping is necessarily their choice nor that it's easy for ADHD kids to just go to sleep. It is not easy! Turning their brain off at night is most probably the hardest thing they do all day.

WHAT WORKS BEST … Let their parents know if they are struggling to stay awake in class. If falling asleep is the problem, recommend the parents ask their GP for melatonin.

Advise the parents that they need to do as much as they can to calm the child's brain down before they go to sleep. Sleep hypnotherapy really works. Aromatherapy diffusing through the night. Mobiles or pretty lights on the ceiling.

And if a child arrives in the morning with black rings under their eyes and yawning, go easy on them. Odds are they've had a bad night and would've much preferred to stay in bed but their parents have dragged them into school.

They may be feeling extremely rough and fragile so look out for tiredness in your ADHD students and be extra gentle with them on those days. Also expect them to be emotional. Being tired very often makes ADHD kids overly emotional.

Important stuff I want to remember:

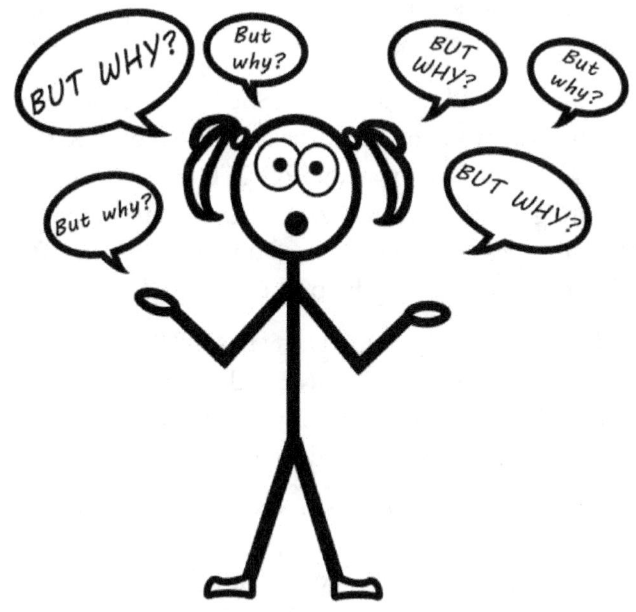

WHEN THEY ALWAYS WANT TO KNOW 'WHY?'

This is a nice easy one to understand even if this constant questioning has been doing your head in up to now.

It is dead simple. An ADHD brain is inquisitive. It doesn't just do something because you're telling it to do something. It wants to know WHY?! And if you can't give a jolly good reason WHY – guess what? That ADHD brain is very probably not going to persuade itself it should do it. Whatever 'it' is.

The best example of this trait I can give is mock exams. You know, those pretend exams you have at school before the actual exams! A lovely, placid and academically bright ADHD girl client of mine (destined for A levels and university) put the fear of God into her parents after taking her mocks, so by the time I met her the family were already in crisis.

Daisy, fifteen, had horrified her teachers by putting her head on her desk and SLEEPING through all her mock exams. The school was worried and perplexed, her parents in full-on panic mode. But within one therapy session, Daisy and I had worked it out.

There was just no point was there? She didn't understand WHY they were important. It suddenly clicked: I had felt EXACTLY the same way at fifteen! What was the POINT of mocks?! They didn't mean anything. Didn't count towards anything. There was no REWARD for passing them. She didn't understand WHY they mattered. Neither had I. So why bother?

We sorted this one out by giving Daisy her OWN reasons for trying at the next batch of mocks. She would do her best in each subject to gauge for HERSELF how much work she needed to do before the actual exams. It worked! She'd found her reason 'why'.

This is an often-overlooked trait of ADHD. But it is a powerful one and can have a huge bearing on an ADHD child's behaviour. Unless there's a very good reason WHY something should be done, the ADHD brain will struggle to motivate itself to do it.

The other huge point to make here is that until you give an inquisitive ADHD child an answer, they aren't going to let it drop. And believe it or not, this isn't them being difficult on purpose. It is their brain that won't let something go until it can make sense of whatever it is asking. They don't want flannel. They don't want fobbing off. They just want the TRUTH. Right now. Quick. No sugar coating and no hanging around. Give them that and they'll be off and running. Until the next time.

However exasperating it is to keep answering the constant WHY question, if you give them the true answer quickly, you'll be surprised how soon they let it drop. And always keep answers positive.

Example:

Child: 'When is it break time? I'm bored.'

Teacher: 'Not for twenty minutes. Get on with your work.' (Negative)

Child: 'That's ages. I don't want to wait that long and this is SO boring.'

You have just given them a reason for a potential meltdown. Or at least not much enthusiasm to carry on working.

Better response: 'Very soon now. Almost there. If you just finish off that last question it'll be break time – plus it's PE next so no more writing today.' (Positive)

This way the child not only knows WHY it's not break time yet but also what to do to make it come quicker AND the knowledge that there's even better things coming. A little adrenaline shot for their reward-seeking brain.

You'll be staggered at the difference in how the ADHD child receives these two different messages.

TOP TEACHING TIPS … Don't ever answer a why question with 'just because' or 'because I said so' or 'because I'm your teacher and you'll do as I say'. Recognise it's a genuine need to understand the importance/relevance/reason for something. All that will happen, by not giving a quick and truthful answer, is you risk a lot of whingeing and moaning and in the worst cases, a physical reaction or a meltdown.

WHAT WORKS BEST … Always give a reason or an explanation. Don't be vague or noncommittal. When an ADHD child asks you a question they need an answer. Always phrase it positively. Remember, their brain is reward based. And don't change or not stick to what you've said! That's unfair (as far as an ADHD brain is concerned), and is going to inflame our heightened sense of justice.

Important stuff I want to remember:

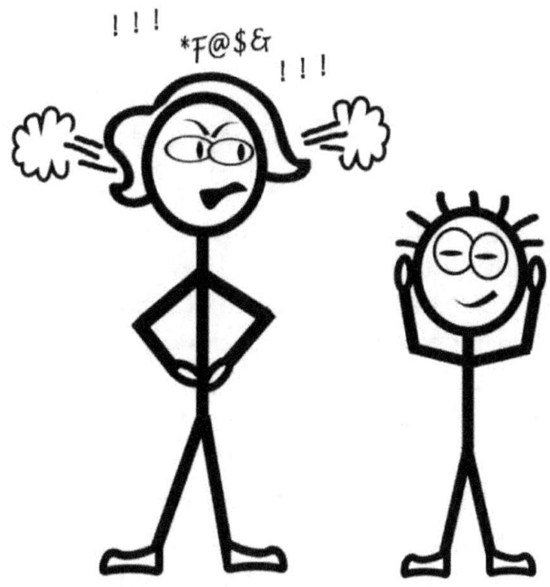

WHEN THEY WON'T DO AS THEY'RE TOLD

This will come as a shock, but there will come a day when your perfectly behaved student, possibly even your bright-as-a-button star student, will suddenly rebel, leaving you speechless when they resolutely refuse to do whatever it is you've just asked of them. In fact, you'll be so shocked, I guarantee you'll ask them to do it several times more, yet there isn't even a slim chance of it happening.

This child hasn't suddenly been replaced overnight by a demon child, but their ADHD HAS just kicked in! There are lots of traits that feed into this 'not wanting to be told what to do'. It could be any of the following ADHD traits and most likely a combo of all of them:

- feeling that we know best

- always wanting everything our own way

- not liking being told what to do

- struggling to interpret instructions and directions

- lack of motivation (especially if something is routine or boring)

- procrastination (unless it is very exciting with immediate reward)

That's quite a mixture to be going on in any child's ADHD brain and at some stage they are going to rebel and not adhere to whatever you are instructing them to do.

Spare a thought for Mum and/or Dad because this element of ADHD is particularly difficult for parents. I have my own theory on this. I think it is why ADHD children, on the whole, get on much better with grandparents, aunties and uncles and often struggle to get along with parents. If you think about it, it makes complete sense. For a brain that doesn't like being told what to do, the parents are usually the main overseers of discipline, rules, instructions and restrictions. And at school that's you!

My own example is pretty typical. I clashed with my mother on a daily basis because she was the one who was hands-on in bringing me up. My father, who I only saw part-time, was much easier to get along with – partly, I now believe, because he was ADHD himself but also because, only seeing him once a week, there was no discipline involved. It was all FUN with dinners out, bowling, swimming, cinema. With my brain being suitably entertained and not controlled, I was probably easier to have around.

It certainly felt easy from my point of view. No constant nagging and boring discipline like at home. It also helped having a stepmother who worked at Mars and brought home selection bags of sweets every week, which I was allowed to eat to my heart's content. No relaxed indulgences ever happened in my own house.

I also had a fantastic relationship with my nan, who never told me what to do, how to behave, how to speak, how to sit, how to eat, or the thousand other things my mother constantly threw at me in a bid to bring me up properly. This led to a long-term, smouldering resentment of my mother. She didn't have the benefit of knowing I was ADHD, so treated me like a neurotypical child and I was anything but.

Luckily, you are better informed. You (hopefully!) know who in your class has ADHD, so I can tell you how to get the best out of them. There are some very cool tricks I have learnt by handling my undiagnosed ADHD niece from when she was just twelve months old. And this works with all kids and teens with ADHD, without a shadow of a doubt. It is very simple and you might think it is so simple that it isn't worthwhile – but trust me on this. This is crucial information if you want ADHD kids to do anything.

1. Ask. Don't tell. If you ask an ADHD child if they would like to finish their history assignment before break you are going to get a much better response than if you say, 'You're not going to break until you've finished that.' Instantly, the child's hackles will be up because they are being told what to do. Reframe it as a question and there will be no irritation.

2. Give choices. I've used this one and it works. When my four-year-old niece didn't want her dinner, I gave her three options. One was to eat from a tray on the sofa, the second was to eat at the kitchen table, and the third was to eat at the dining table. She looked at me murderously, knowing she had been caught out but also realising that I had just put her in charge. I'd sought her opinion, which made her feel important and she therefore made a decision – passing on her wisdom, as she saw it!

   So if you really want a child to finish a piece of work try, 'How would you like to get this finished? We can either do it together after school, or you can take it home and finish it tonight or we could meet for half an hour before school tomorrow?' Put the child in charge of making the decision, while always making the choices ones that suit you. You'll be surprised how affable and amenable they become when they are 'in charge' and not being told what to do.

3. Negotiate. The ADHD child will have reasons why they are against doing something. It is up to you to find out what those reasons are. Some may be unreasonable, but some may be just. For example, if a child has social anxiety or any of the other coexisting conditions of ADHD, there may well be a genuine reason why they don't want to do something. So it is definitely worth opening up the conversation around what it is you want them to do and why they are not keen to do it.

It is going to be a very rare ADHD child who doesn't give you this problem. At its earliest, this trait will kick in from the age of two but if you're lucky it might not arise till puberty. But, trust me, it is going to feature heavily in the teenage years.

The tone of your voice is also very important when you speak to an ADHD child. Any sign of anger, irritation, bossiness or unreasonableness will be met with frostiness at the very least and, at worst, anger and meltdowns.

If you keep your voice soft and ASK things, keeping it POSITIVE and QUESTIONING rather than telling, you are always going to get a much better response than somebody who is barking orders.

Shouting or raised voices is a real no-no with ADHD kids. In my experience about eight or nine out of ten ADHD people also have sensory processing disorder. I do. So when anybody shouts, my irritation/anger levels shoot from one to a hundred instantly. I've never punched anyone in my life but shouting makes me instantly vicious!

For parents (always) – and potentially/possibly teachers too if you can arrange it – when getting an ADHD child to do anything becomes a real struggle, you might want to consider a reward system. This 'not wanting to be told what to do' is one of the very best reasons to implement a reward system. Remember, tiny adjustments can have a major impact. So if it takes the promise of an early break to get the child to do something, don't be frightened to use it!

ADHD kids are strong willed. So be prepared for the battle they will put up BUT know that negotiation and them feeling they are in charge is key to solving this as quickly as possible. Options work. Open discussion works. Understanding where they are coming from and listening to their reasoning works.

Ultimately you do have to get them to do whatever is needed and these really are the best ways of going about it.

TOP TEACHING TIPS … Avoid shouting, getting visibly angry or irritated when an ADHD child won't do something. Don't try to force them into action by shouting louder or humiliating them.

WHAT WORKS BEST … Try to get underneath what is really going on. What is the problem? Why do they not want to do it? Do they have a genuine reason? Is this an indicator of an undiagnosed comorbidity? Are they struggling to interpret instructions or directions? Do they not understand what is required of them and are avoiding humiliation by instead refusing to do it? Dig until you find out.

Important stuff I want to remember:

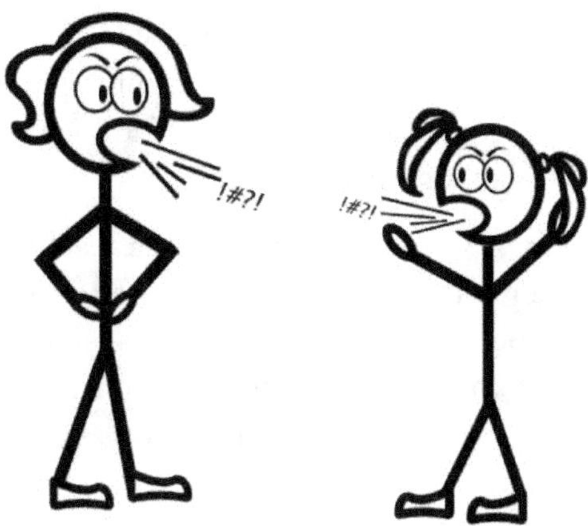

WHEN THEY ANSWER BACK AND ARGUE WITH YOU

This is another very big problem and potentially the reason you bought this book in the first place! Answering back to teachers, arguing relentlessly with parents, brothers and sisters, and seemingly being able to start a fight in an empty room is an absolute ADHD trait. And there is a very good reason for it.

Before we get to that point, just a bit of empathy from me to you. It is a very rare ADHD child who doesn't like an argument. This usually starts from the age of about eight or nine. I have seen children as young as five give their parents a right mouthful if they are told off, but generally it is when puberty looms that the problem really starts.

At the very least an ADHD child will be deemed to have 'attitude'. I had this levelled at me from the age of about twelve. If only I could change my attitude everything would've been okay – apparently! But I couldn't. I wasn't purposely behaving in any way. It was my natural demeanour. But it seemed to offend people deeply. Even my nan, who I worshipped and adored, told me I 'made her feel an inch tall' when I was about twelve. I was mortified as I didn't ever want to hurt her, but this apparently was all down to my attitude.

You might get away with an ADHD kid just having this sort of 'screw you' attitude, but often that's not enough for a spiky ADHD teen. More often they will argue the toss about anything and everything and will leave you exasperated by their seemingly never-ending enthusiasm for an argument.

And believe me, just because you are their teacher don't assume this means they're going to respect you. As far as ADHD children (and adults) go, respect has to be earned. This isn't hard. If you talk to them politely, don't shout or humiliate them and listen to what they have to say, they are going to respect you and your life is going to be so much easier.

There are a lot of ADHD traits that feed into this 'knowing best and letting you know that', but first let's talk about the brain. An ADHD brain gets adrenaline from fighting. It loves not only banter but a proper full-on fight – and the more you engage or argue back, the more it is going to carry on.

Have you ever remonstrated with an ADHD kid for having to have the last word? I can almost guarantee you have! That's because their ADHD brain will not let it go. If you say something to them, they just have to say something back.

So what you need to do is be one step ahead. Remember that their ADHD brain is seeking adrenaline and it can get that from having a good old shouting match with you or anybody else. If your aim is to get the shouting to stop then you've only got to do ONE thing. It is a very simple thing but it is also the hardest to do in the circumstances. That is to say your final piece – and then walk away.

Try it. It is very powerful. If you think it is difficult for you, learn from the young offenders I worked with in prison who I told to walk away from baying crowds, desperate to see them fight. It nearly crippled them doing it the first time, but with practice they could walk away and without exception they all then realised the power they had gained by doing this.

That power really is in your hands and if you can say what needs to be said calmly, clearly and with no hint of anger and then walk away, the ADHD child's brain will soon lose interest in fighting or answering back as it is not being fed the adrenaline.

It is a good idea to tell class mates to do exactly the same. Putting it simply, the more you engage with ADHD fighting talk, the longer you are going to prolong the episode.

A lot of the time you will find this arguing talk is due to the ADHD trait of having a heightened sense of justice. If anything is deemed to be unfair you can guarantee an ADHD child is going to become outraged. They will go from zero to a hundred in two seconds flat if they feel they are being taken advantage of or that things aren't fair.

The other trait at play here is the fact the ADHD child will always think they know best and that they are always right. Remember this is not a choice. It is the way their brain works.

Something else to be wary of is the fact that an ADHD child's brain won't let something drop. Unlike a neurotypical brain, which can just let something go, this never happens in an ADHD brain. If something isn't right or fair or just, the ADHD brain will keep ruminating and overthinking it and will absolutely not be able to let it go.

If this is a really serious problem it might be an idea to suggest to parents they look into oppositional defiant disorder (ODD) and pathological demand avoidance (PDA). Kids with these conditions take arguing to a higher level. I often wonder now if I would have been diagnosed with ODD myself; any sign of incompetence and I leap on people from a great height!

Your goal is to be in a position where you're not giving the ADHD child anything to shout about. This is a real challenge. Here are some of the things to look out for because these will really ignite an ADHD brain:

Never humiliate an ADHD child. I mean NEVER. Not in fun and definitely not seriously. Humiliation is taken very badly by an ADHD child and they can see humiliation where you might not. I will give you an example. The father of one of my clients wanted to put a video of him as a baby on social media. Despite my thirteen-year-old client begging and pleading for him not to do it, the video went on YouTube. Suffice to say my client's right foot then went through the television screen, and it was only then that the parents realised how humiliated he had felt.

Be very careful how you talk to an angry ADHD child. Anything that can be perceived as humiliation, mickey taking, or putdowns are going to get an immediate angry reaction.

The good news is for most ADHD kids, by the time they hit their very late teens or early twenties a lot of this rage has subsided. They will have mimicked from neurotypical friends how to behave in public and will have learnt how to manage their anger. For a small minority, however, it carries on being a problem in adulthood and an even smaller minority end up in prison because of it.

TOP TEACHING TIPS … Don't do or say anything intentionally that is going to unnecessarily wind up an ADHD child. Remember that they can't regulate their emotions, they have a heightened sense of justice and their brain feeds off the adrenaline of fighting.

Simply speak to them with respect and you'll get it back.

WHAT WORKS BEST … Be mindful of how you talk to them. Don't engage if they are wildly flinging argumentative phrases at you. And make other children in their class aware of the consequences if they purposely annoy an ADHD child.

Understand their ADHD jangling hormones might make them appear antsy and irritated for the whole of their teens. They can't help their attitude so don't take it personally.

Important stuff I want to remember:

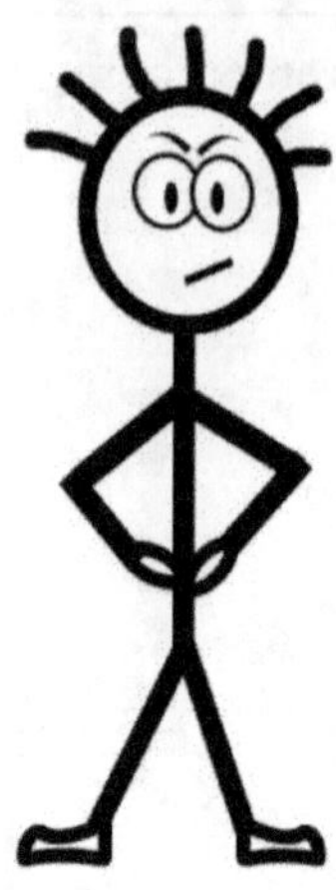

WHEN THEY THINK THEY KNOW BEST AND WANT EVERYTHING THEIR OWN WAY

This is a biggie. If you've been teaching an ADHD child, you'll have very probably encountered this already.

But did you know it is an actual ADHD trait? Thinking we know best and wanting things our own way is the way our brain is wired.

Bearing in mind I wasn't diagnosed ADHD till I was fifty-one, my mother spent decades calling me a 'control freak' and saying, 'WHY does everything have to be YOUR way?' Now we know! It is not the easiest trait to have and it does lose us friends. You can imagine how the ADHD child in a group of mates, always wanting to do joint activities the way THEY want, would drive the others nuts. It is also not easy for parents. And definitely not for teachers!

How do you handle it, particularly with pre-teens and teens who haven't yet developed the awareness to know how to tone down this side of their personality?

Firstly, don't argue. This will get you nowhere except into a heated argument or, worse, a meltdown. Whatever the ADHDer has just decreed as law, such as, 'I'm never doing geography homework ever again,' don't retort with, 'I think you are, young man. You'll do as I say.' That won't get you where you want to be. Instead, ask questions.

Yes, you did hear me right. Asking questions in a genuinely inquisitive manner (not sarcastically or patronisingly) will do two things.

1. It will make the child feel important. Remember, they like to feel they're in charge, so you are straight away playing into that element of their brain.

2. It will make them feel like their opinion matters. So they will gladly share their wisdom with you. This will get them talking. As they start communicating calmly, that is your chance to help them to see things from another angle – yours.

So here's an example.

ADHD: 'I'm never doing geography homework again.'

Teacher: 'Oh. Can I ask what's the problem?'

ADHD: 'I don't get it.'

Teacher: 'What is it you're not getting?'

ADHD: 'I just don't understand what he says. So I can't do my homework 'cause it makes no sense and I haven't got a clue what he wants me to do.'

Teacher: 'Ah, I see. Sometimes Mr Smith gets very passionate about his subject and maybe he isn't explaining things clearly enough to you?'

ADHD: 'Yes. I would do it if I knew what he meant.'

Teacher: 'I'll have a word with him. Make sure he sees you to explain anything you're not clear on whenever he gives out homework. I'll ask him if he will send you the PowerPoint of the lessons by email as well if that will help? Don't worry, it won't be in front of the other kids; I'll make sure he talks to you discreetly.'

ADHD: 'Thanks. I wish more teachers understood, like you.'

Hey presto. No meltdown. No argument.

See. It's easy! Well, it is if you remember to question rather than tell.

Another thing to bear in mind is that often we DO know best. Why? Because our brain can often see the quicker or easier way of doing something. So if an ADHDer is proclaiming that something can be done better – give them the chance to explain how. Again, ask questions. Give them the opportunity to express what's going on in their brain.

Listen. Hear. Discuss. Negotiate. Compromise. Agree.

In that order.

And remember that once something has come into an ADHD brain, it has to come out. We can't just put the idea to one side and move on. Our brain won't let us. So let them speak. Let them get it all out. Then with gentle questioning (with no hint of sarcasm or belittling), discuss whatever it is they're thinking.

ADHD kids will push you. Some push blooming hard. I've seen it in therapy. They have no concept they could be wrong. And no concept that your opinion might be the more reasoned let alone right. Your questioning skills may need brushing up on. Google 'motivational interviewing'. It is handy in situations like this.

The more you battle an ADHD child the more aggro you'll have in your life. Their brain is powerful, especially during puberty when their hormones are all over the place. Their strength at wanting their own way could shock you.

TOP TEACHING TIPS … Don't ignore their views. Don't ridicule or mock them. Don't tell them to stop talking or say, 'NO,' without them being given a chance to speak.

WHAT WORKS BEST … Ask questions. Listen intently. Take them seriously. Show that you are genuinely interested. Gently encourage them to look at things a different way. Ask if there IS another way of looking at it. Hone your negotiating skills!

Important stuff I want to remember:

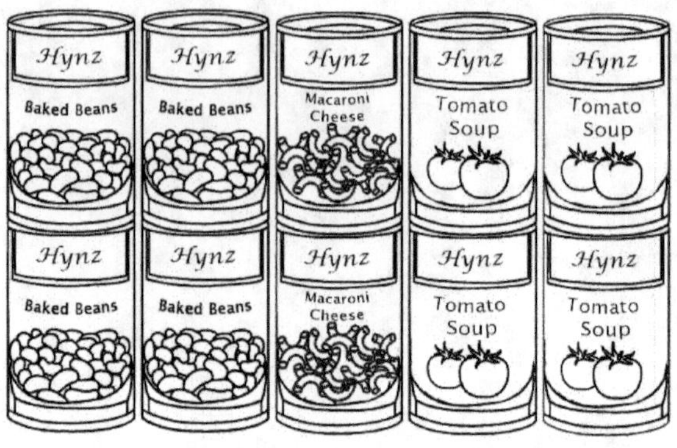

WHEN THINGS HAVE TO BE JUST RIGHT – AND PERFECTIONISM

It is quite common for some people with ADHD to have perfectionism. This might seem like a massive contradiction if you've only seen whirlwind ADHD kids operating in disorganised chaos, not seeming to give a toss about anything, let alone where it goes!

I've no idea what percentage of ADHD people also have perfectionism, or anankastic traits as it can also be called, but it is quite a chunk and most of these appear to be girls and women. I have it myself. Fully diagnosed and all.

Perfectionism isn't to be confused with OCD. While admittedly there is a lot of overlap, full-blown OCD will always have negative thoughts attached, such as, 'If my tins aren't all facing the front and up the right way, my dog will get run over'. Perfectionism doesn't have the negative thoughts attached. But that's not to minimise the effect of it. It can have a huge impact on someone. If I explain how it affects me, it might help you understand the magnitude.

For me things have to be exactly 'right' or I can't function. 'Right' can be different things to different people but for me it is all to do with cleanliness and tidiness. A psychiatrist once asked me how I would feel if all my tins in the cupboard weren't facing the front and up the right way. I couldn't answer. He saw the look of abject horror on my face. Eventually I mumbled out, 'It just wouldn't ever happen.'

As disorganisation is a widely known ADHD trait, how can ADHD then be linked with perfectionism? I've my own theory on this. I worked it out from my own ADHD brain! I believe some of us hate the natural chaos and mess we create, BUT because we aren't naturally neat and tidy, we have to work twice as hard to keep things in order. From this constant battle – and I mean 24/7, year in, year out – comes the mania that leads to perfectionism.

Here is one example. I have to be on top of my washing. If the pile of laundry gets too high, I literally can't function. I feel overwhelmed and like I'm falling behind, which leads to feeling sad, hopeless, useless and incompetent. It feels like I will never be on top of it all, or my life, again. Because I don't want to feel like this, I'm a woman possessed with emptying her laundry basket on a crazy, stupid, regular basis. Bingo! There you have it: perfectionism.

If an ADHD child is displaying stubborn behaviour and insisting on things being 'right', look deeper into why. I'll give you some examples of how this might present.

- Not wanting to go to school because one item of clothing isn't right.

- Not wanting to do homework because the computer/textbook/pen isn't right.

- Needing to re-start a piece of work because they've made one mistake.

- Needing a new notepad because they've made a stain on the cover.

- Not wanting to eat because something isn't right. 'Because a pea touched a fish-finger,' is one of my favourites!

- Not wanting to play football because they've brought the wrong shorts.

- Not wanting to go to certain places or events because the journey/venue/catering/music 'isn't right'.

Remember, perfectionism in ADHD is born from anxiety, so try to be as understanding as your health and temper will allow. Much as you might want to strangle an eleven-year-old who now won't eat his fish-fingers at lunchtime because they have the wrong fish in them (also true story) after having happily eaten them before, understand for him it is now not a possibility. He really is not just being difficult.

Perfectionism is not something anyone would choose. I'd pay good money to get shot of mine. So do some research on the subject if you think your student may have it.

TOP TEACHING TIPS … Don't keep pushing them if they really are insistent that they can't do something. Don't humiliate them, make threats or chastise. It won't work and will only increase their anxiety.

WHAT WORKS BEST … Ask what the problem actually is. Help them identify it. They might not even really know. What would make things right? What needs to change for things to be right? It is often something quite minor. Try to understand where they're coming from.

Avoid a stand-off. It won't get you anywhere. Communication and understanding will. And if it is a minor change, like needing a new pen or a new notepad because they've ruined the first, your and their life will be easier if you allow it.

Important stuff I want to remember:

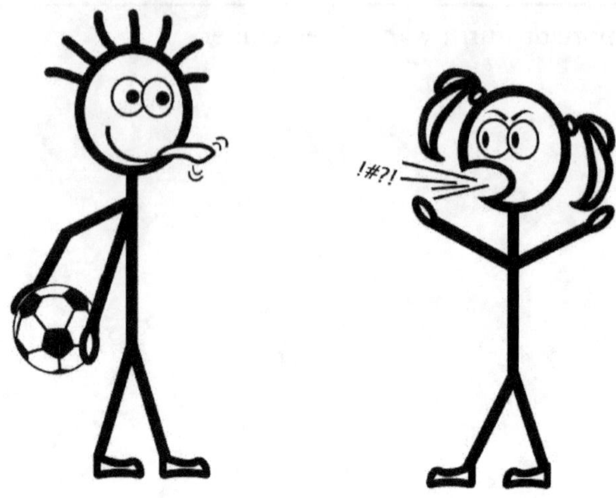

WHEN THEY WON'T SHARE

This is a lesser-known trait and doesn't apply to all ADHD children. But the ones it does, it is usually quite severe and can cause problems, especially when young.

I've done a lot of research on this and I'm not absolutely sure where it comes from. But my guess is it is possibly the ADHD child liking to keep everything under control. We do like to be in charge and to have things our own way so sharing can be torturous.

And I believe perfectionism often plays a part in not making it easy for us to share. In this context for me it means that unless everything is 'perfect' (and that means having everything to myself and everything under my control) I'd rather not do it or have it at all.

It could also come from the trait of our heightened sense of justice. As soon as we start to share something, we can start to feel that the other person has an unfair advantage. And we never, ever, like that.

I remember from childhood that if I was told to share anything, I would rather not have had it at all! And this has stayed with me to this day. It doesn't come from petulance; it comes from genuinely wanting something all to myself or I would rather not have it at all.

Anxiety may play a part. I remember a sense of dread that, if I was sharing, I wouldn't get a fair deal.

I see many families with siblings where sharing becomes a problem. The ADHD child wants to do things their way, at their speed and the way their brain wiring thinks is better. This can clash with neurotypical children and also another ADHD child, who might see things even more differently! This will be exactly the same at school, so be aware that any games or activities where an ADHD child is expected to share might result in a moody strop and an 'I'm not doing it.'

At home Xbox- and PlayStation-type games can become a living nightmare if siblings are supposed to share. It is far better to split the time up and let each child have a certain time doing the activity than to get them to share it.

The same at school. Make very sure any activity that involves sharing is managed so the ADHD child knows they are getting a fair deal. An idea I love is if there's anything that needs splitting in two and sharing – let's say a cake – get the ADHD kid to do the cutting in half. Then the other child chooses which half. You can bet your life that ADHD kid's precision when cutting anything in half will be spectacularly accurate! Put the ADHD kid in charge; they'll ensure things are fair!

TOP TEACHING TIPS … Try to avoid situations where an ADHD child has to share if you can see it really makes them uncomfortable or angry. When it's unavoidable, make clear plans in advance. Wishy-washy arrangements make an ADHD child anxious they'll miss out.

WHAT WORKS BEST … Making sure any situations where they are expected to share are very clearly managed. Make the boundaries and expectations from each child abundantly clear. Don't leave any grey areas. The ADHD child will need to know they're getting a fair deal to relax enough to partake.

Important stuff I want to remember:

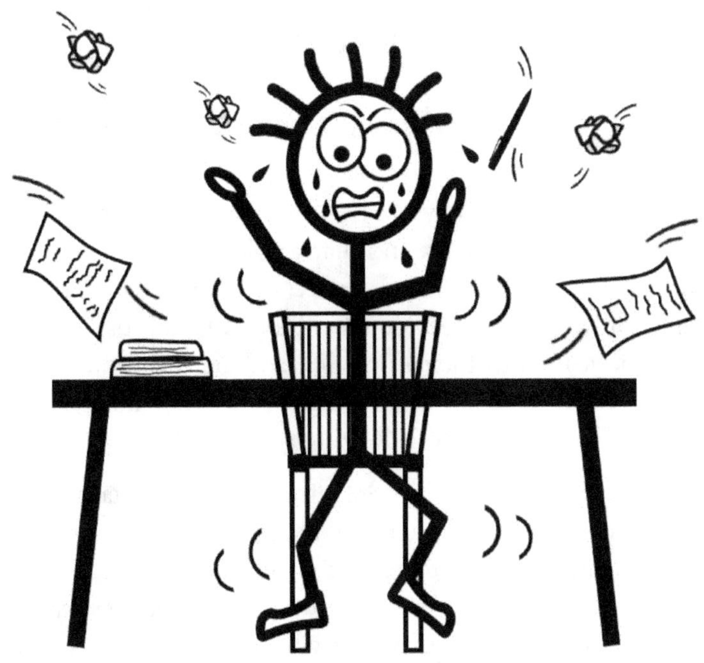

WHEN HOMEWORK BECOMES A NIGHTMARE

There are two types of ADHD kids when it comes to homework: me and the rest! Or that's how it would appear. I was radically different to most ADHD children in that I wanted to get my homework done and out of the way the minute I walked in from school. It can't just be me, though; there must be other ADHD kids like this.

I remember rushing through the front door after school and heading straight to my bedroom and cracking straight on with all the homework I had been set. I couldn't enjoy my play time until the work had been DONE. I did it all in double-quick ADHD time and was chapters ahead of my peers in all the subjects, according to my mother.

If your ADHD student is one of THOSE kids, you won't have too many problems. I was like this right through from age five to seventeen. It never changed. Even at counselling college, decades later, I still did my homework and got rid of it as soon as I possibly could. I think this is possibly due to that perfectionism trait and the dreaded fear of overwhelm. If I could keep on top of things by doing them quickly, I had much less chance of being overwhelmed and feeling out of control. Being in control has always been very important to me.

However, it is highly likely your ADHD student doesn't have this attitude towards homework and that would be far more common! For most, homework is pure torture: an irritating and intrusive continuation of what they've been loathing all day. To have schoolwork 'leak' into their home life and encroach on their own time is a major frustration for a lot of ADHD kids. And this particularly relates to ADHD boys.

ADHD girls, generally speaking, fall into the category that thinks, 'I'll comply even if it annoys me, and it'll be last minute – probably at midnight or on the bus into school'. Boys often – not always, but definitely often – are more likely to think, 'I'll find every excuse under the sun not to do it. And if you force me, then watch me kick, scream, shout and generally make your life hell for BULLYING me into doing something I REALLY DO NOT WANT TO DO'. It is this last challenging lot we will deal with here!

Firstly, please remember this child could well be dealing with one or more undiagnosed coexisting conditions of ADHD that is making studying way harder than it should be. I was. It took till I was fifty-six to work out I had, and get a diagnosis for, dyscalculia. Never heard of it? Neither had I at school. But it is more commonly known as 'the numbers version of dyslexia'. And it is the reason I failed my 12+ exam. One of the traits of dyscalculia is not being able to solve problems. So that was my grammar school education up the spout.

It was also the reason I received a 'U' for maths and an 'A' for English at O level (thanks Bucks Education for not picking up this was clearly indicative of a learning disability). Bear this in mind if the child is bright and having absolutely no issues with English and history, but flounders dismally with maths, economics and any subjects involving numbers. Also look out for signs of dyslexia.

Especially in girls. It is very common. Also, dysgraphia which makes putting words down on paper difficult.

Don't assume the paediatrician who diagnosed the child's ADHD necessarily picked up on any of these coexisting conditions. I've met countless children (and adults) where the diagnosis of ADHD has been given but the comorbidities haven't even been investigated. And it is important. Massively important. The amount of adults I have met who have had their lives crippled by undiagnosed comorbidities is heart-breaking.

The rejection sensitive dysphoria (RSD) part of the ADHD child's brain is not going to want to be humiliated for being slow or getting bad marks. So they'll cover up. Usually by mucking about or kicking off. Case in point – maths was where I was at my most witty and entertaining, where my 'clown of the class' ADHD trait was most prominent. I couldn't get to grips with what was being taught so entertained/stimulated my brain myself this way instead.

So look at the subjects where the ADHD kid is struggling, because these are the classes for which you won't be getting homework handed in. Which subjects do they 'hate'? Which homework do they want to tackle least? Which homework never appears or has been eaten by the dog? Then dig deeper to find out what's really going on.

Once you're sure there are no learning disabilities affecting the ADHD child's ability to do homework, we can assume it is any one of the myriad ADHD traits that are coming into play. Take your pick!

- procrastination
- lack of motivation
- not being excited by it
- boredom
- not liking to be told what to do
- not seeing the point
- having no respect for the teacher, or what they require of them.

Any or all of these could be coming into it. It doesn't really matter which ones are impacting the child; all that matters is what you do about it. And these are my top tips.

Firstly, put the child in charge. Let them decide when and where they are going to do their homework. Would they prefer to do it during school hours? Some would rather skip lunch break if it means taking no work home at the end of the day.

If they choose to do it at home but it's still not happening, start gently probing and liaising with their parents. It may well be that the child needs a quiet place or a low-noise-level place or a place on their own or a place where they can see Mum or Dad. Each child is different. Find out what they NEED and where they need it. And let the parents know that trying this out is definitely worth a go.

Often, life in an ADHD household can be loud and chaotic because, being hereditary, there isn't just usually one person in the family with the condition. So if a student tells you that it's just too noisy at home with Mum nattering constantly on the phone, Dad screaming at the racing on the telly and three younger brothers and sisters squawking, then you need to have a quiet word with Mum to explain that this child really does need somewhere quiet to do their homework.

And if that means going to their nan's, where it's quiet, a couple of nights a week or making some sort of other similar alternative arrangement, help the child make that happen. Their parents may well be oblivious to the problem. ADHD kids are fabulous at not telling parents when they have homework. Trust me, some are masters at it!

If they are choosing to do their homework on the school premises either before, during or after school, until you know and see different, believe the child when they tell you what works best for them. If they say they need music on in the background, let them. If they say they need their headphones on, let them. If like me, they need absolute silence and the door shut and their annoying younger brother kept well away, make sure they are left alone.

If it turns out they were having you on and listening to loud music really isn't conducive to them working well, you will need to gently and with encouragement point out that as yet homework isn't appearing as regularly as you'd like.

Keep it positive! Remember you are always on their side and want the best for them. Encourage them to try alternative environments or stimulation levels. It really is one rule for one and one for another.

I've met ADHD teenagers who flunked GCSEs because they were put in a room with no posters on the wall, so they had nothing to look at to calm themselves down. I've known others fail exams because there was intrusive noise and too much activity.

Most children work best when their homework is broken down into chunks. If they know they have to do thirty minutes' work followed by a cup of tea and some biscuits, they are going to work much better for those thirty minutes than they would have done for forty-five. Encourage parents to structure this with the child, to put alarms either on their phone or an egg timer or something they can see. Usually, an ADHD child can work flat-out for a short period of time as long as it is followed by a break with a nice little reward to look forward to, even if that is just two chocolate biscuits with their milkshake.

When ADHD children are very young, to keep them from being distracted and inattentive, it is usually best if parents or their teacher sit with them while they do the homework. It will be better Mum, Dad or you spending thirty minutes making sure it gets done rather than nagging them for two hours and it doesn't get done.

As they get older, they will want to be more in control, and this is fine but they may well need help with structuring their homework times.

As always, reward systems come into play here. If the promise is they will be team captain next time they play football for the school, as long as they get that week's homework into you by Friday, you'll be surprised how motivated they become!

I've seen parents use everything from 50p a day to a football match ticket for Tottenham as incentives. Whatever it takes it will be worth it, both for their sanity and the kid's education. Something nice to look forward to after homework is a necessity! So if their parents haven't thought about this, and are really struggling to get their ADHD kids to do their homework, mention it to them as something definitely needing to be put in place.

Also worthy of note is that tutors usually work extremely well for ADHD children; these kids thrive on one-to-one attention. It means they can learn at their pace if they are particularly fast or particularly slow, and it is much less easy to get distracted when you are the only one in the room.

I've known many ADHD teens to be falling behind at school and then flourish within weeks of studying with the right tutor. So if a child is really struggling and the parents can afford it, do suggest this to them. It might not have even entered their head as a possibility. It is well worth looking for a tutor who is experienced in ADHD and any other coexisting conditions the child might have. Especially if it is something like autism. The child will hugely benefit from being tutored by a specialist and they do exist.

And for those kids for whom none of the above works (and there are some), is this homework actually critical for their learning? If you believe it is, then is there a different way this information can be presented that would appeal to an ADHD brain? For example could they watch a YouTube video on it, or work on an interactive lesson online, which stimulates them visually? If you are asking for an essay could it instead be a bullet pointed piece to demonstrate their understanding? Or could they make a PowerPoint presentation or something more creative for you? This will ensure the learning still happens in a way that will appeal to even the most homework-hating kids.

TOP TEACHING TIPS … Don't expect an ADHD child to just sit down and do their homework without any fuss on a regular basis. If they've not handed any in, find out why. What's going on? Are they struggling to understand what's required of them? Is the environment at home a problem? Would they rather do their homework at school? How can you best facilitate this?

WHAT WORKS BEST … Ask a parent to sit with them and do their homework with them until they are old enough to do it on their own. Then make sure they decide collaboratively where it's best they do their homework, what environment is going to work best for them, whether they need white noise or complete peace and quiet or music or headphones.

As the child matures, encourage the parents to decide in conjunction with the child the sort of length of time they feel they can study for without needing a break. Make sure those breaks have something nice enough in them for the child to aim for, whether that's a hot chocolate or a cuddle with the dog.

Finally, suggest parents think about having a system that rewards them at the end of the week and the end of the month for such things as doing their homework on the right day, without nagging, and handing it in on time.

And if particular subjects are a problem, encourage the parents to think about some tutoring, even if only in the short term. It can make the world of difference.

Be creative. There are tons of different ways of getting information into an ADHD brain. Staring at or writing words is likely to be the least appealing.

Important stuff I want to remember:

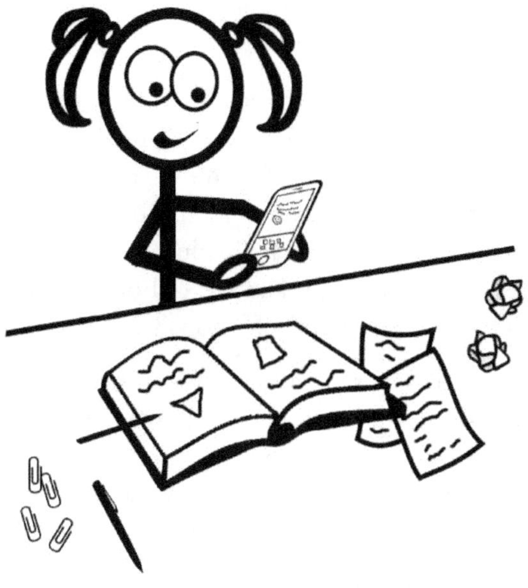

WHEN THEY CAN'T OR WON'T REVISE

Now this is something I think might surprise you. ADHD brains HATE revision! And there's a clue in the word: it is the 're' bit. It means repeat or re-do something. That is never going to stimulate an ADHD brain that only likes NEW and EXCITING activities. So getting ADHD children to revise is going to be one of the biggest nightmares you'll ever have! However, what I'm going to tell you now works, so there is hope!

I could never understand why I couldn't revise. I wanted to revise, I wanted to do well in the exams, and I knew that revision was the key to it. But boy, was it a massive struggle. I couldn't concentrate on the paper; if I'd read something before, it just did not stimulate my brain enough to read it again and my short-term memory was so shocking that nothing stayed in anyway.

So go easy on ADHD kids around revision time. They will be surrounded by classmates talking avidly about how much revision they've done, and the ADHD kid will probably have a ton of anxiety because they know they haven't done the same amount. And it won't necessarily be because they're not bothered. They might be

VERY bothered but just not able to do it. So here are a few ideas that should work.

ADHD brains learn best at the last minute. I actually set my alarm for six o'clock on the morning of my English literature O level to finish reading *Cider with Rosie*. Cramming at the last minute meant I passed – with a C – because my brain took the information in 'in a crisis', when the adrenaline was flowing. I hadn't been able to finish reading it before, much as I knew I should have: those last few chapters just weren't interesting enough for my brain.

ADHD brains work best in a crisis when the adrenaline is flowing. Therefore, an ADHD child is going to learn and store the information much better as the exams get closer. So there really is no point putting a six-month revision plan in place, but there are other things you can do that will help.

ADHD brains need to be stimulated and that means by something new. There are lots of alternative ways of getting information into an ADHD child's brain, but the least effective will be them sitting down looking at text. So it's a good time to get your creative thinking cap on and come up with different ideas. These are ones that I've seen work in the past, but you will no doubt come up with some of your own.

Let's take English as an example. If a child is studying a play, arrange a school trip to see a live performance of it where possible. Outdoor performances where you can take a picnic are always a good bet because they can fidget/move without being told off and nibble food and drink to keep their hands occupied. Take a school trip to the cinema to see a big screen version of the play. If there's an audiobook version, see if the school library can invest in a copy. If budgets don't stretch that far, mention it to the parents. Ditto the film if there is one. If they're studying Shakespeare, and it is within the school's budget, visit Stratford-upon-Avon and the William Shakespeare museum.

Try to stimulate their brains around the subject. ANYTHING is going to be better than just reading the plain text.

Think about the subjects they are studying. There is a huge number of museums/places to visit that might be relevant to other areas of their learning. And there will be crossovers. So a trip to a museum might help with science as well as geology.

Because their ADHD brains are likely to accept information as exams get closer, put a structure in place that means they have plenty of time for study in the last couple of weeks before the exam. That's really when most of the information will sink in.

Advise the parents not to go organising social events, take them on holiday or plan lots of play dates around this time. It really will be in that last two to four weeks that the adrenaline will kick in and much more of the information they are learning will stick.

Rewards work when trying to help children to revise. They learn best in short bursts with a reward at the end. So when the adrenaline is flowing and they are in learning mode, make sure you structure it so they get regular breaks and a reward at the end.

At home that reward might be fish and chips. At school maybe break time starting ten minutes early. I still remember the little thrill that ran through me when we were 'let out early' and break went from fifteen to twenty-five minutes. An ADHD reward-driven brain is easily pleased.

Another highly successful tip is to write facts on Post-it notes and have them visible, whether that's in their bedroom, on the fridge, in the dining room or where they study. Helping them at school to write up facts, dates, and information they need to learn on Post-it notes and then taking them home with them really works. Because the notes are brightly coloured and in small segments, the ADHD child is much more likely to remember what's on them. So if they're studying in the kitchen, lounge, bedroom or dining room they can take the relevant Post-it note with them, and bring them back into school easily if needed.

Another tip that works is testing a child. If you remember that ADHD brains like to win and rise to a challenge, asking them to do some revision in class and then you testing them on it is a brilliant way for it to stick in their brain. So regular quizzes in class on subjects they are learning will massively help them retain the information. I used to love being 'tested'. And ironically getting a question wrong, and then finding out the RIGHT answer fascinated my brain enough never to get that wrong again.

All ADHD kids are different when it comes to the best environment to revise. I could only do it in complete silence. However, I know of many children who need white noise or the television on in the background before they can concentrate enough to take in information. If a child is struggling to revise it might be worth mentioning these options to parents.

And if motivating an ADHD child to revise at all is difficult then remind them that with ADHD in adult life, they won't like being told what to do and they will want to have all the choices. If they don't get the grades they need to get into college or to study whatever they have chosen, all those choices get taken away. Get across to them that as much as you know revision is difficult, it is a necessary evil if they want to have all the best choices later on in life.

TOP TEACHING TIPS … Don't assume revision will be easy if they put their mind to it or that it's just a question of them sitting down and looking at a book for long enough. It really isn't and that won't work. Be mindful of their self-esteem. Just because they aren't brilliant at revising doesn't make them any sort of failure. Be sure they know that.

WHAT WORKS BEST … Be creative. Think of different ways of getting information into an ADHD child's brain. Think cinema, movie, theatre, events, museums, YouTube, googling: any different way of presenting that same information to the child which is exciting and not boring.

And remember they are going to revise best at the last minute so don't panic them six months before exams. Start talking to them about it six weeks before!

Important stuff I want to remember:

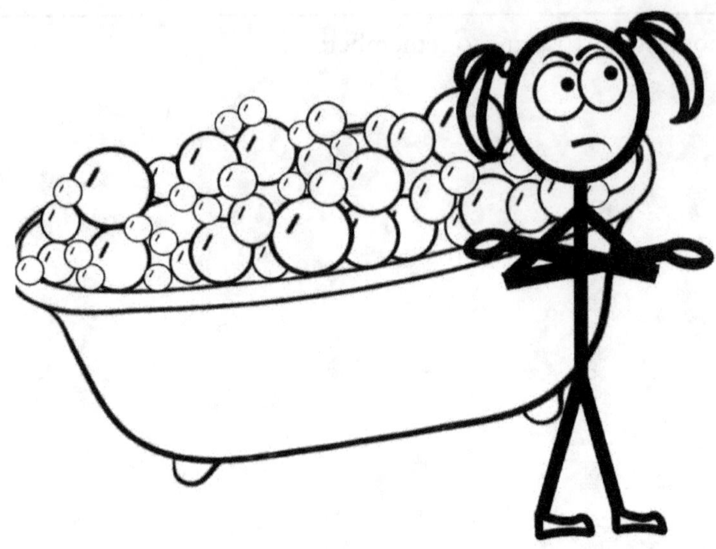

WHEN HYGIENE GOES OUT THE WINDOW

For those of you who have no experience of this yet, it might come as a surprise. But I can almost guarantee at some point most ADHD early teens are going to get very bored with ablutions and not bother with even basic hygiene!

There is one very simple reason for this. Getting showered or bathed, hair washing and getting dressed is incredibly boring. And mind-numbingly repetitive! ADHD people really don't like doing anything over and over again, especially if they can't see the point. So having regular showers or baths and washing their hair, and even brushing teeth, can be seen as really unnecessary and dull.

I am the most fanatical clean freak there is now but during my teens I went through a classic ADHD stage of deciding cleaning my teeth was unnecessary. The next time I went to the dentist I had to have FOUR fillings, which hurt like hell, and from that moment on I've brushed my teeth twice a day. But it was several weeks, if not months, when a toothbrush didn't go near my mouth!

Equally, bathing was terribly boring for me. So there was a time, when I was about twelve or thirteen, that I'd run a bath, perch on a little chair next to it reading a book and swish my fingers in the water to make my mother think I was in the bath. I don't think this went on for very long before comments were made that I was a bit on the whiffy side, and I must've decided to start washing again.

But even to this day I find the daily shower and hair wash the most monotonous and boring part of my day and I've always said if I could pay somebody to do it for me, I would. And I've met more than one adult ADHD client in therapy who has admitted they can go for days without showering because they find it desperately dull.

So expect your ADHD students to go through a patch of either not showering, bathing, washing hair or cleaning teeth. It really is to be expected and my advice would be to put up with it for as long as you can without making a scene; usually they will decide for themselves that greasy, unwashed hair makes their head itch or their face will become spotty and that will be the wake-up call to reintroduce washing into their daily routine!

If it gets seriously bad and other kids in the class are refusing to sit near the stinky kid, then it might be time to have a discreet word with the parents.

For those of you with ADHD kids of your own, here are a few extra tips.

Remembering that ADHD kids don't like being told what to do, you have to make 'keeping themselves clean' their idea, not yours.

You could start by casually mentioning how nice people's teeth look on the television, how nice their favourite singer's hair looks, and any other gentle, subtle hint you can come up with to make them realise their chosen way of avoiding cleanliness isn't going to result in the same.

The key really, to make hygiene more exciting, is to give them a reward. 'Exciting' could mean a waterproof radio in the shower or a waterproof television near the bath. Or make it so they don't get their tea or bedtime snack until they have showered. A reward after showering/bathing is a simple but effective way of getting them in the bathroom.

Another good way is to buy them gifts of luxury designer aftershave or perfumes – sports stars' and celebrity ones. You know the sort of thing. Encourage them to emulate their idols, be that by using body sprays, aftershaves or shampoo.

And very occasionally it can be sensory issues that can be the problem. So dig deep. Do they not like the feel of the shower on their skin? Some can feel it is like knives stabbing them. Or does the feel of the toothbrush on their teeth literally cause them pain? A lot of ADHD kids don't like the taste of mint. There are alternatives for all these issues once you've managed to uncover what they actually are!

TOP TEACHING TIPS … Don't think a stinky ADHD teenager is anything unusual. Accept that it is just a phase and the vast majority of them grow out of it quite quickly.

Sit them near an open window and if things don't improve reasonably quickly, arrange for a discreet chat with the parents and give them some of the advice that you have read here.

WHAT WORKS BEST … Advise the parents to talk to them about ways of making washing more exciting. What would work for them? Would they like a radio, television or something else in the bathroom to liven things up a bit?

Explain to the parents that you understand that washing and showering is boring and it doesn't stimulate their brain. So they need to look for ways together to make this activity more fun with perhaps a reward afterwards.

Important stuff I want to remember:

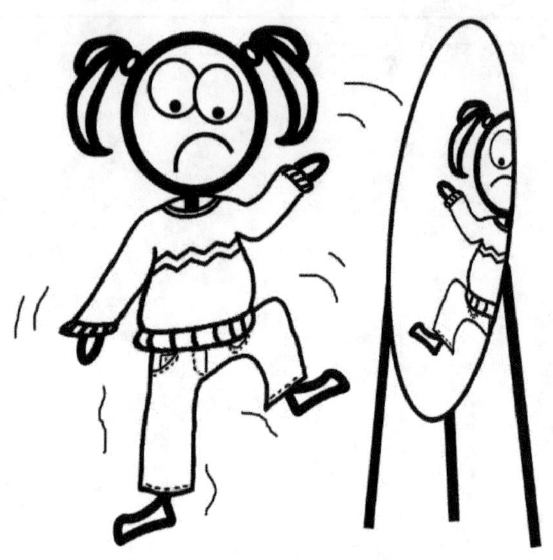

WHEN THEY START GETTING FUSSY
ABOUT CLOTHES

One of the coexisting conditions of ADHD, and probably the most common, is sensory processing disorder (SPD) and this is usually why clothes may become something of an issue with ADHD kids!

Most ADHD people have a problem with what materials touch their body. The vast majority of ADHD kids and adults I know won't tolerate anything scratchy, itchy, fussy or tight around the neck or clothing that clings to their body. So if ties are obligatory at your school and the ADHD kid is always pulling theirs away from their neck, loosening the knot and trying to undo the top button of their shirt, don't be surprised.

Conversely I have met the occasional ADHD child client who wears clothes up to five years younger than their age because they have to have all clothing stuck like glue to their body. These kids can't bear anything loose and flapping so they will wear underpants and trousers for children five years younger to make sure that everything sits incredibly snuggly on their body.

However, nearly everybody else with ADHD wants to wear denim, cotton, jersey and loose-fitting clothes. And an extraordinarily large number of ADHD people don't like wearing shoes. Most report that they would spend their lives barefoot if they could. I'm sitting here barefoot writing this!

I'm a classic example of SPD and I remember reacting very violently as a child to my mother trying to put me in a mohair jumper and a scratchy yellow poncho; thankfully not at the same time. And polo-necks clinging to my throat made me feel like I was choking. To this day I will only wear denim, cotton and jersey, and I cut every label, hanging strap and spare button out of clothes before they even make it out of the shopping bag and into my wardrobe.

The chances are high that your ADHD student, too, will have issues with clothing. SPD is something you might want to look into as so many ADHD kids have it and it can affect ADHD children in a ton of different ways.

Some not only have issues with touch but also smell and taste. Certain smells do make ADHD kids feel sick and they might not be exaggerating. Like, I wasn't exaggerating when I told my mother the smell of cucumber sandwich spread made me feel sick. Ten minutes later when she was clearing up the evidence of that, she got it!

Clothing labels are usually a massive no-no for ADHD kids. They rub on and irritate the skin and at least 90% of ADHD people cut out their labels before they put their new clothes on. So if an ADHD child approaches you yanking the back of their jumper away from their neck or pulling their trousers away from their back and begging you for a pair of scissors to cut the label out, it will be because their parents have forgotten to cut that particular one off.

SPD will most likely be the overriding problem ADHD children have with clothes, but there might be other factors that need to be taken into account.

One is fitting in at school. The ADHD child will probably already be conscious of being different and standing out because of their ADHD, so the one thing they won't want to do is stand out because of their clothes or shoes. If they tell you they want to wear certain things a certain way because they will feel more comfortable, let them – as long as it's legal and stays within the realms of decency of course!

Another ADHD trait that can play a part here is perfectionism: wanting everything to be exactly right. Some even quite young children will get very bolshy about clothes or shoes not being right. I vividly recall my three-year old niece wailing, 'I'm not comfy! I'm not comfy!' because I hadn't lined up the seam of her tights on her tiny feet as she wanted.

Some will be overly particular about there being no stains or marks on their clothes or shoes. Particularly trainers. With teens, white trainers will become their parents' own personal nightmare. If there is so much as a tiny stain, they will likely find themselves being asked for new ones. And if anybody should be as gung-ho as to drop anything on or damage any item of clothing or shoes an ADHD child particularly loves, expect an explosion because you will get one. This will probably be a mixture of perfectionism and SPD. One blob of tomato ketchup on their jumper will ruin their day. And it really will, so don't ridicule them for it.

Something else to bear in mind is that an ADHD kid's body can often be warmer than those of other children. For starters, because they move around so much, are restless and constantly on the go, they can get much hotter and sweatier than neurotypical classmates. Also, if they're on medication this can raise the body temperature slightly, so if your ADHD student really doesn't want to wear their blazer in March because they are too hot, don't insist they do. It is not going to kill them and it isn't worth the risk of setting off World War Three just because it's 'school rules'.

Also be wary of hats and caps. I remember my junior school uniform hat had an elastic string that went under my neck. That string irritated the life out of me and I was constantly pulling it away from my neck. So if you can collaboratively come up with a way that keeps the child's uniform in line with other students but takes their SPD into account, the child will thank you.

A quick mention of self-esteem here. It is accepted that ADHD children have lower self-esteem than neurotypical children, so if an

ADHD child insists something makes them look fat or uncool or is too babyish for them it really will be easier to just swap the item for something else rather than risk them doing what I did. For two whole years of my school life, I hated the shoes my mother made me wear so much that I used to change into plimsolls at the beginning of the school day (behind the bike-shed so nobody saw me) and wear them all day and every day. The hated shoes were old-fashioned and guaranteed to have led to name-calling and bullying, which I was terrified of. It was easier to put on my plimsolls and carry my shoes around with me all day. Granted the 'cool kids' at my school were wearing four-inch platform shoes and my mother was right in that she didn't want me breaking my ankles, but it was hell for me standing out as 'different' in a tough school environment.

TOP TEACHING TIPS … Try not to assume an ADHD child is just being fussy, or difficult, or making a big deal about nothing if there's something they just won't wear. SPD is a very real condition and gives a lot of distress to people if not recognised.

WHAT WORKS BEST … If the child really isn't happy with one item of their uniform or any sports kit, school play costume or anything else you are asking them to wear, don't just force them to wear it. If they hate something, find out why – without judging. Try to work with the child so that you find a compromise that suits you both.

Important stuff I want to remember:

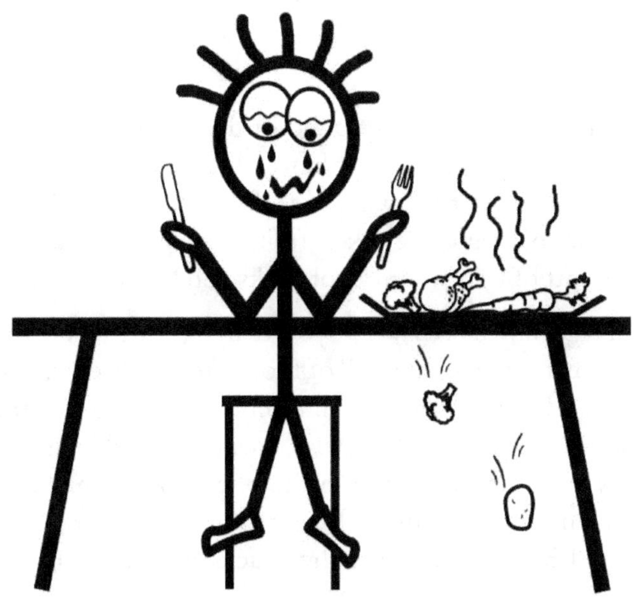

WHEN FOOD BECOMES A PROBLEM

There could be a lot going on when an ADHD child starts having problems around eating, and these range from the mildly irritating to the majorly worrying. So tread with caution before you start pushing them to finish everything on their school lunch plate and telling them, 'There are starving children in Africa who would give their right arm to eat those Brussels sprouts.'

Some of us with ADHD have more of a compulsive eating problem. When I was a child practically nothing filled me up. I remember my mother angrily telling at me at the end of dinner, 'Well go and have a slice of bread then!' whenever I whinged I wasn't full. She was thinking a slice of bread was the LAST thing I would want. She thought I was after more pudding. This saw me swiftly exiting into the kitchen and relishing eating bread and butter because I really was still hungry.

So the first thing to look out for is compulsive eating. An ADHD child's brain is always telling it that 'nothing is enough'. It needs more. When they eat a meal they aren't listening to their tummy and realising that it has had enough, let alone waiting the twenty minutes recommended to see if it is actually full. Not a hope. Instead, an ADHD child's brain is saying, 'This is nice, this is yummy; I want more.'

One of the best ways I have found of dealing with this within the home is having a tin, box or drawer that is full of little healthy snacks the child can have whenever they feel they are hungry. I'm talking about oat bars, rice cakes, fruit, small packs of raisins – you know the sort of thing – or carrot sticks and hummus in the fridge.

It doesn't go down well when you deny an ADHD kid food, but making sure it is the 'right kind' of food is relatively easy. Make sure there's lots of variety and it is all healthy and don't give them any restriction on it. If you restrict, all you will get is a child like me who was forever sticking her hand in the biscuit barrel, grabbing what she could and foraging for food in the kitchen in secret. Far better that a child has access to healthy snacks whenever they feel the need.

At school I know this isn't so easy. If the child has school dinners they should be able to fill themselves up at lunchtime but might need to bring a couple of healthy snacks for morning and afternoon breaks. And don't be surprised if an ADHD child wants to bring their own packed lunch in. Often they will have so many restrictions around food that they will want to bring their own in from home.

If a child is at the other end of the scale and gets 'funny' around food there could be all sorts going on. Some ADHD children are very fussy about how their food is presented. I've met ADHD kids who won't have baked beans on the plate because they 'leak' into other food. I've met ADHD kids who will only eat peas if they're in a separate bowl. I've met ADHD kids who won't eat anything with gravy because they like to pick their food up with their hands. And I've met an awful lot of ADHD kids who can't stand sauce of any kind – even tomato ketchup!

And I've met kids who, like me, are very funny about the texture of food. I can't eat nuts because they taste like cardboard or raisins, sultanas or currants because they are all wrinkly and I can't stand the wrinkly texture.

Sensory processing disorder will almost always give kids issues with food.

An ADHD child may not even know what's going on themselves, so some gentle exploration with them will go down very well when it comes to finding out what they will and won't eat. They might not even know why they don't eat certain things. I certainly didn't realise it was the texture of things I had a problem with until I was much, much, older.

For other ADHD children it can be the smell of things, the look of things, the colour of things and whether or not they are crunchy or smooth. There is literally no end to the issues an ADHD child might have around food that you might not have even thought of. Even as an adult the smell of goats cheese turns my stomach so much I'll move tables if someone nearby orders it on a pizza.

And if a child has the coexisting condition of ASD, it opens a whole new door to even more problems on a much grander scale.

Another major problem can be sitting at the table to eat when you have ADHD hyperactivity and restlessness. It is not just the child being difficult if they can't sit still. It is this strong and chronic desire to move and DO something that means they can't just sit still. If this really is a problem for them then you have lots of options but do take it seriously into account.

You might decide that an ADHD child can leave the table whenever they need to as long as they come back to finish their food before the end of the lunchtime break. You might agree they can have a ten-minute run around the playground in between dinner and pudding. Come up with options that suit you both.

Don't allow other students to have their dinner time ruined by forcing an ADHD child to sit at the table when they really can't. Take their ADHD into consideration and make alternative arrangements. This isn't 'giving in' to them not sitting at the table. It is taking their condition into account and making reasonable and acceptable adjustments that work for you, your ADHD student and all the other children.

Something else that might be going on is overwhelm. Big dinners can be overwhelming to an ADHD person. I remember Sunday roasts being plonked in front of me and feeling a kind of overwhelm and exhaustion just looking at it. And I was a compulsive eater! For kids who aren't really interested in food this is just going to be a mountain too big to climb.

What works much better for ADHD children when it comes to food is variety. I know this is more difficult at school but at home I strongly recommend you consider having tapas-style dinners: several items in bowls in the middle of the table from which a child can dip in and out as they wish. The ADHD child likes variety and this is going to appeal much more than one big plateful. You can make it as healthy as you like but try not to give them a massive plate with just three items on it. Bowls in the middle of the table with half a dozen items is going to go down much better, especially for finickety eaters.

At school one option might be giving them a couple of side plates or bowls and allowing them to split things up so it's not quite so overwhelming. Another benefit is they can arrange their food so things don't touch, if that is a problem for them.

We also need to take into account eating disorders. I have met both girl and boy ADHD teenagers who have developed binge eating, anorexia and bulimia. It is not hard to see why some ADHD children go down this road. If you consider that low self-esteem and anxiety are usually part of the ADHD condition, it is quite easy to see why eating can become disordered. As a counsellor I've seen a wide variety of eating issues including avoidant/restrictive food intake disorder (ARFID).

Keep a watchful eye on an ADHD child's eating patterns, particularly as they hit puberty. This is when the ADHD overthinking, low self-esteem, anxiety, compulsive and impulsive brain activity can impact on their eating.

ADHD medication can also severely affect appetite. A lot of ADHD children (and adults) report pretty much losing their appetite while their medication is working. This means an ADHD child may have very little appetite, if any, during the day but will want to eat like a horse in the evening.

Rather than trying to force a child to eat three similar sized breakfast/lunch/dinners in a day, far better is to let them have a protein-based breakfast in the morning and another small amount of protein at lunchtime. Not only will this help the medication work better, it is also healthy.

You will need to liaise with their parents about this. If they are hardly eating anything at lunchtime but the parents tell you they are eating a big breakfast before they take their medication and then a big dinner at night when it's worn off, you shouldn't worry too much about them not eating much at lunchtime. The focus then is to ensure they are getting most of their nutrients in their breakfast and dinner.

And although it's tempting, don't comment on what is in their lunchbox. A child who is restricting food intake may have high-fat food in their lunchbox purposely to boost calories. Hearing one critical comment from an adult can set them on a dangerous path. If you have any concerns speak to the parents.

If an ADHD child really struggles with appetite, then protein bars and protein shakes can be a good replacement lunch, as long as they are getting a very well-balanced breakfast and dinner.

TOP TEACHING TIPS … Don't expect an ADHD child to sit at the table and eat their dinner with no issues at all. Ever. It is unlikely to happen. Disordered eating and eating disorders go very much hand-in-hand with ADHD. Anything from anorexia to bulimia and everything in between could feature, so keep an eye out and flag up anything unusual to their parents.

If they are having school dinners, don't force them to eat food they say they have a problem with. You'll end up with a child who, like me, more than once vomited all over the school dining table when I was forced to eat food I just couldn't stomach.

WHAT WORKS BEST … Be watchful of binge eating, compulsive eating or restricted eating behaviour. Find out from their parents if the ADHD child is on medication. Make sure they are getting a healthy balanced breakfast and evening meal and be prepared to negotiate what they will eat at lunchtime. They may only need a protein shake or a protein bar or a very small amount of protein at lunchtime.

Important stuff I want to remember:

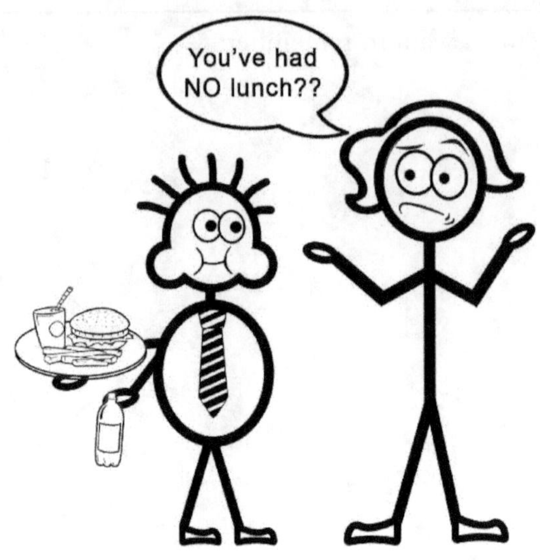

IF THEY START LYING

The youngest ADHD child I have actually witnessed lying was four years old. You might have your own horror story of lying starting younger than this but four is still incredibly early. Much more likely is that an ADHD child will start to slip in the odd lie by the age of around six or seven. This will pretty much always be them getting themselves out of a hole, or lying about having done something they consider boring like their geography homework.

Lying comes quite naturally to most ADHD kids and I know it can be a major problem in some families and for their teachers, because if they're lying at home, odds are they are at school, too. So let's first tackle why ADHD kids may lie and then we'll go into what you can do about it.

Life can be very boring when you are an ADHD child. I remember lying to liven things up and make things a bit more interesting. I also lied to get what I wanted. Particularly in the food department. I became very adept at putting my hand in the biscuit barrel, under the beady eye of my mother, and in one swoop pulling out four biscuits instead of one.

My lies were all little and harmless (apart from my guilt over one poor librarian) but I've worked with hundreds of ADHD young offenders who lie through their teeth. So much so I think most even believe their own lies. So if we first accept that, if an ADHD kid is lying, they are probably doing so for one of these reasons:

- boredom and the irritation that comes with it

- wanting to shock or push boundaries

- wanting to be the centre of attention

- wanting to get away with not doing something boring like homework

- for personal gain such as, 'I've not had a second helping,' when they are on their way to collect their third pudding

- needing to liven things up or make a story more dramatic

- because they've genuinely forgotten and think they are telling the truth.

And, of course, it could be a combination of any or all of these. The first thing you need to do is understand it's quite normal behaviour for a young ADHD person to lie. That's not saying you have to accept it, and yes we do need to do something about it, but don't think it is anything out of the ordinary, because it really isn't.

I strongly suggest you don't turn it into a game of cat-and-mouse and try to catch the ADHD child lying. All that is going to do is feed the adrenaline in their brain and make them even more determined to get one over on you.

So how do you tackle it then? My answer is to first make it very clear to them how important the truth is in life. Perhaps interweave this into your lessons, always remembering that the ADHD children won't be thinking of the consequences of lying.

Give them examples of how people lying in history has caused problems. Find really dramatic examples. Well-known people who have been sent to prison for anything that involved lying. There are a good few infamous ones to choose from!

Your ADHD students in particular need to know that lying is never right and that however bad the truth is, it is always better than a lie. Something that works very well is giving them a certain amount of time to admit the truth. If you suspect something is a blatant lie, it is very unlikely the child is going to admit it immediately. They won't want to be humiliated, causing rejection sensitive dysphoria (RSD) to kick in. But if you have a '24-hour rule' whereby they can come to you with the truth and there won't be ANY repercussions, you will find a lot of ADHD kids will come to their senses when the heat of the moment has passed. A surprising amount actually. And surprisingly quickly. I think this is where our heightened sense of justice does us some good.

It is a very sensible idea to allow them to communicate this to you in any of several ways. You can put some good systems in place whereby the child has a route OUT of their lie, back to the truth. Otherwise, sometimes we feel that we can get backed into a corner and we have to lie just to get ourselves out of it.

Make it very clear to the child that lying is NEVER the right route, that honesty and the truth is ALWAYS the best way, and then make it easy and accessible for them to do that. It will mean giving them lots of choices as to how they admit the truth. For starters they aren't going to want to do it in front of classmates because that will be humiliating. So you need to find a confidential way they can. This might mean they leave a note in an envelope on your desk, are allowed to email you privately or can have a confidential one-to-one chat. I strongly suggest you decide this collaboratively with the child once you realise that lying has become more than a one-off for them. If they have been involved in choosing the ways they can communicate the truth to you, they are far more likely to use them.

And when the child does tell you the truth you need to make a very big fuss about it. Praise them, thank them, enforce how important the truth is and how they made the right decision. The more you do this the more likely they are to admit the truth the next time.

This really is one of the ADHD traits I firmly recommend you nip in the bud as soon as possible. I've seen far too many ADHD boys in young offender institutes who are adept liars. I'd go so far as to say pretty much everybody is in prison because they lie. There aren't many honest criminals kicking about. I've also worked with ADHD teenagers of around seventeen and eighteen who have been getting into hideous problems with the law because of lies. Lies really do need to be stopped in their tracks as early as you possibly can.

There's no need to panic and think this is anything unusual for an ADHD child but also don't ignore it. Don't humiliate them or chastise them without trying to get to the bottom of the problem. That won't help improve matters and will probably just lead to more lying.

TOP TEACHING TIPS … Don't accept lying, cover up for them or hope they'll just grow out of it. Don't call them out for lying in front of their classmates. This will most definitely bring on RSD and humiliation, which is ten times more difficult to bear when you are ADHD. Don't punish them for it because this behaviour is very much linked to their ADHD. But deal with it as quickly as you possibly can.

WHAT WORKS BEST … Use the phrase 'not telling the truth' as it sounds a lot less harsh than 'lying'. Speak to them confidentially when you know or suspect they've not been truthful.

If their parents are not already aware, explain to them that you know that not telling the truth can quite often feature in ADHD people, especially when they are young, so they need to let their child know that lying when you have ADHD is quite common. This is very important because when they have been caught out for lying they may well think, 'I must be a terrible person; I'm different to everybody else and I'm hopeless'.

Collaboratively come up with ways they can tell the truth and come clean after the event. Make it very clear that all will be fine if they tell you the truth within a certain period of time. Praise and thank them for their honesty when they do.

Important stuff I want to remember:

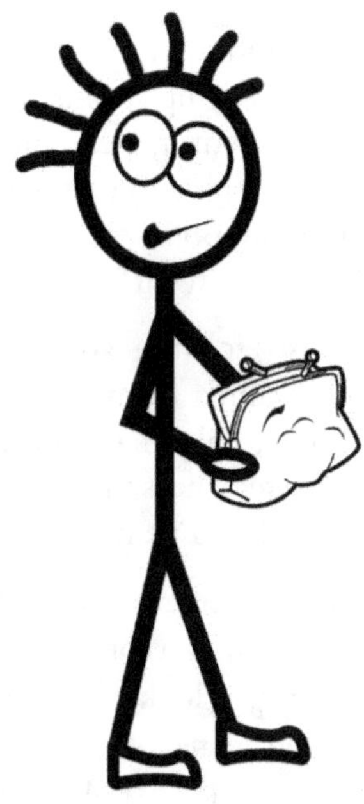

IF YOU FIND OUT THEY ARE STEALING

Not all ADHD kids pinch things but a lot of them do. I don't consider myself a criminal, but I was quite a prolific thief in my early teens. Not only was I swiping sweets from the sweet shop, I was also on a very regular basis filching money out of my mother's purse. This was always for food, and nearly always when we went swimming with the school and I wanted to get my fair share of snacks from the vending machine afterwards.

I remember thinking I was a real smarty pants because I only took coins that wouldn't be noticed. So for example if she had three 50p coins I would only take one of them. This was when I was round about twelve years old. I cannot recall ever being caught, but that could be my dreadful memory! Anyway I know it went on for quite a long time and I considered myself very clever for getting away with it.

The reason why ADHD kids steal things is, I believe, primarily because of two traits.

1. Our impatience and wanting things NOW. We steal because we don't want to wait, to save up money and then buy something in three months. If we want it, we want it NOW. So stealing is the obvious answer. And if we see other kids having stuff, like I did at the swimming pool vending machine, we don't understand why we can't have it NOW either.

2. I think we do it also for the adrenaline rush. There is an incredible buzz to be gained from stealing things. I had it in my early teens. (Thankfully, I also had the fear of God put into me by the police who visited the school to tell us the impact of a criminal record on our life. I've never nicked anything since!)

As with all things ADHD, you might find this a minor problem with your ADHD students or a major one. I've actually worked with families who have had to put locks on fridges, kitchen cupboards and even bedrooms. One teenager was so notorious for swiping anything, the family had to keep their handbags locked in their bedrooms to be sure he wouldn't be dipping into them.

Some ADHD kids have a real problem with stealing. They literally can't walk past anything that catches their eye without grabbing it. This can get them into big problems in shops. They will see something on the shelf and have it in their pushchair from the age of three! Honestly. From as young as that. But usually stealing doesn't become a problem until about the age of eight and, as with me, it is highly likely to ramp up as puberty hits.

Once you've realised your ADHD student is stealing, it is time for THE VERY SERIOUS TALK. Rather than telling them off in front of classmates, sit them down when things are calm. These are the messages you need to get over:

- You're not judging them for stealing and you understand that this is almost definitely part of their ADHD. But together you do have to do something about it.

- Ask them to explain to you what it is they get from stealing. Are they doing it purely for the excitement or is it because they want things they can't afford?

- This is something you need to tackle together because you don't want this impacting the rest of their life. You are ON THEIR SIDE.

- Explain to them how easy it is to get a criminal record.

- Explain the likelihood of them needing a bigger buzz, leading onto more serious stealing and more serious problems for them.

- Do your research beforehand as to which countries they won't be able to travel to if they have any sort of criminal record. Explain how this can seriously impact future travel plans.

- Talk to them about how they will be limiting their career choices.

- And if they're still not getting the message, tell them how carrying on with such behaviour is only ever going to end up in one place – and that place is prison.

If it is money they want, and often it is, talk to them about different ways of earning money. Perhaps their parents could utilise their skills around the house or garden? Or get them washing cars for neighbours?

If they are at the right age, suggest a part-time job. Encourage them to start earning money early because ADHD kids are usually driven, they want things, but you need to educate them on how working for it is the much safer and more satisfying route.

Many of the young offenders I've worked with in prison have started stealing in their early teens because they wanted the latest trainers, tracksuits and devices. Not one of these boys had a Saturday or part-time job. I, however, started working at the age of twelve and had my own money from then on. So if you can instil a work ethic into an early teen you've much more chance of them not pilfering.

And don't forget the ADHD inability to think of the consequence. This is the serious bit. You can almost guarantee they won't have thought of the consequence of impulsively popping something off the shelf and into their pocket. Without terrifying them, you need to get the message into their brain that one quick action could have serious repercussions for the rest of their life.

Again, ideally, interweave this into your lessons so the ADHD kid doesn't feel singled out. But hopefully, like when the police came to my school, it will resonate with them when they realise that the short-term thrill is going to massively impact their choices as an adult.

Important stuff I want to remember:

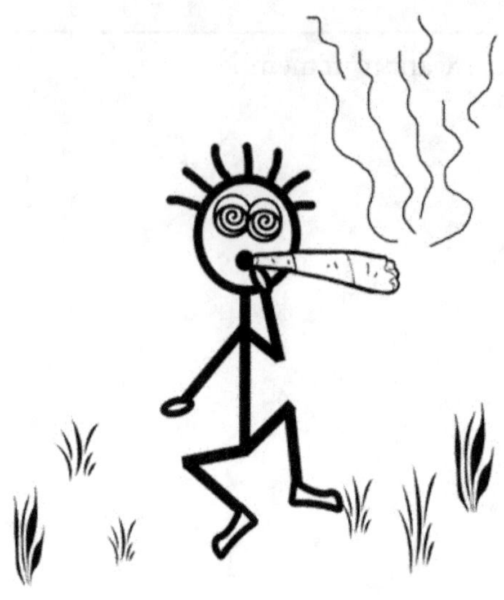

IF YOU SUSPECT OR KNOW THEY ARE USING CANNABIS

In my experience the vast majority of teenage boys with ADHD use cannabis to a lesser or greater degree. I don't have a clue on the percentages (and even people purporting to can't possibly know the true figure), but from the thousands of ADHD teenagers I've worked with, I would say around 80% of the boys have smoked weed in their teens. A dramatically lower percentage of girls use it, but it is still not uncommon. There are two overriding reasons for this. All of them tell me that it calms their brains and helps them sleep.

However, the last thing I'm doing is advocating the use of cannabis because I've seen the damage it does. I've seen both the short-term paranoia and the long-term brain damage, so please don't think I'm any sort of advocate for the use of cannabis. And I have never, ever, used it myself! But I have sat in front of trillions of boys in their teens and twenties who tell me they use vast amounts of it. A lot of them do it every day; those who don't use it as much usually have it late in the evening because it helps them switch their brain off so they can sleep.

There's lots of information out there for teachers and parents worried about a child smoking weed so I'm not going to regale you with all the facts and figures and whether it leads on to harder drugs. Instead, I am going to tell you how best to deal with an ADHD teen (sometimes even younger) who is using it. Obviously your school will have their own rules and regulations around this but they very probably won't know about it from an ADHD perspective. So I'm going to tell you how I advise parents to deal with it with ADHD kids because most of this information will be useful for you as well.

Most importantly, if they are hiding it from their parents and you have found out, the parents need to know as soon as possible. And they in turn need to talk to the ADHD child about it sooner rather than later. But that doesn't need to be in any sort of judgmental, shouty or angry way. Instead, parents need to sit down and have a grown-up chat with them about why they are using it, what it does for them, where they are buying it (which is crucial) and always, ALWAYS check that they are not giving it to their friends or selling it.

Giving it to friends means they could be arrested for supplying and selling it obviously makes them a drug dealer. You would be staggered by the amount of ADHD kids who don't realise this. They genuinely think they are being helpful buying it for their friends and not making a profit when they give it to them. These 'helpful' teenagers don't realise that buying cannabis off someone and then passing it onto their friends at cost price means they are any sort of drug dealer! The police view it another way and I've met many, many ADHD boys in prison for supplying or dealing cannabis.

The reason parents need to know where they are buying it is for the child's own safety. I could tell you a good few hundred stories of boys who have found themselves in major trouble by using dodgy dealers and stories of parents having to get involved in paying dealers off.

There is no correct legal way to buy cannabis, at least not in the UK, but you can make sure any child is doing it as safely as possible. If they're buying it in public or by visiting a crack-den, where harder drugs are being dealt, this is obviously riskier than buying it in somebody's private home.

I strongly recommend parents don't panic about this situation but understand it is quite typical for ADHD teens to experiment with weed. Parents need to try not to judge nor make demands. The more you demand an ADHD kid stop immediately, the harder they are going to dig their heels in. And then they will start doing it behind parents' backs, which is much more worrying. Remember, ADHD kids like pushing boundaries, don't like being told what to do, think they know best and want everything their own way. So the more you tell them this is a bad idea, the more they are going to do it. And the more likely they are to experiment with harder drugs just because they enjoy pushing those boundaries!

Everyone involved is far better off opening up the communication around cannabis, understanding how the child thinks it is helping them and trying to find alternate ways to achieve the same thing. So for example, if they are using it to help them sleep, look at different ways of helping without the use of cannabis.

It is often a sign that an ADHD child isn't on the right ADHD medication if they are smoking cannabis extensively. If they are on the right medication, they shouldn't have the need for anything else to calm their brain and if they aren't sleeping there are legal avenues to go down that are far less dangerous than using cannabis.

Do your own research on the damage weed does and communicate this in a positive way with your students. Rather than proclaiming, 'If you touch any drugs you're going to end up on heroin and dead in a ditch,' which isn't terribly inspirational, try, 'I'd hate for you to end up with chronic paranoia, so let's do our best to keep you properly educated and usage as low as we can.'

TOP TEACHING TIPS … Don't panic when you find out any ADHD child has traded the sweet shop for the local drug dealer. It happens. A lot. Whatever your school policy is, and whoever you have to report it to, make sure you let them know that this child has ADHD and that the use of cannabis is extremely common with ADHD kids.

Understand that they are self-medicating their ADHD, like thousands have before them and thousands will after them. Accept that it is the most common way for ADHD teenagers to stop their racing brain and to get to sleep at night.

WHAT WORKS BEST … Let the child know that you are aware and what steps you have to take next. Open up the lines of communication and keep them open.

Make sure their parents know where they are buying cannabis and ensure they are smoking it as safely as possible. Encourage them all to become educated around the effects of weed if they aren't already. Advise their parents to be honest with the child's ADHD paediatrician or psychiatrist about the level of use because it will affect the impact of their ADHD medication. And don't forget to signpost parents to their local Drug and Alcohol Service, who will be able to offer them free help and advice. I've been with clients to numerous of these and even worked in one for eighteen months and the amount of support you can get from a good service is phenomenal. Obviously they vary but it's definitely worth investigating what your local provider can offer.

If school policy allows, include in lessons how as teens they need to make grown-up decisions on whether they are prepared to risk chronic paranoia, psychosis and potential long-term brain damage by using cannabis. Even the most stubborn of ADHD teens doesn't usually want this and if you 'are on their side', helping them make the best decision for them, even the most determined weed user will see the reality of its long-term use.

Important stuff I want to remember:

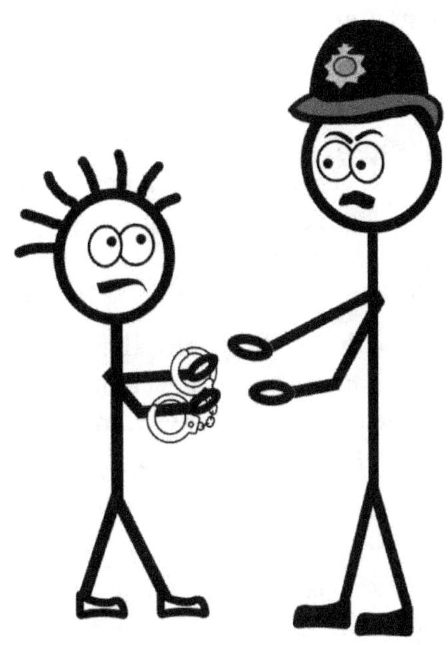

IF THEY START GETTING IN TROUBLE
WITH THE LAW

There is a chance that your ADHD students are going to come into contact with the police when they are in their teens, and sometimes pre-teens – a higher chance than with neurotypical kids. It's not unheard of for ADHD kids to start pushing boundaries and pursuing risky, thrill-seeking behaviours, at times getting perilously close to committing crimes of criminal damage, threats to kill, and affray/GBH/ABH from the age of eight-ish onwards.

Some of this activity may well be at school. So the first thing we need to remember is which ADHD traits feed into this potentially criminal behaviour and to stress that getting the police involved is often not necessary. If you can contain the incident and deal with it internally you are saving that child from stepping on to the horrendously slippery slope and potentially a revolving door of juvenile/young offender/adult prison life.

So at the first sign of any criminal behaviour, stop and think. Is this behaviour or incident connected to their ADHD? Odds are high it is.

I'll give you some examples:

Threats To Kill

ADHD traits possibly feeding into this are impulsivity, not thinking of the consequence, heightened sense of justice, emotional dysregulation, overly sensitive.

Criminal Damage

ADHD traits possibly feeding into this are impulsivity, not thinking of the consequence, rejection sensitive dysphoria, emotional dysregulation, hyperactivity, internal motor, pushing boundaries, risk-taking, thrill-seeking, heightened sense of justice.

You see where I'm going with this? I could go on but I suspect you can already see why so many ADHD traits can be responsible for ADHD kids getting into trouble. And how easy it would be to just pick up the phone and let the police sort it! But unless it's serious crime – I'm talking knives, weapons of any kind and sexual assault type – I'd encourage you to deal with these issues internally and with the parents involvement where necessary.

ADHD kids get angry. They get frustrated. They get bored and their brain constantly pushes them to look for more exciting things to do. Of course this is going to lead them into some dodgy situations. Here's a few examples of teens I've counselled and the problems they've found themselves in:

- Fifteen-year-old boy angry at how his ex-girlfriend was being treated by her new, abusive, boyfriend. ARRESTED FOR THREATS TO KILL.

- Thirteen-year-old boy out with friends became involved in a fight. ARRESTED FOR ARMED ROBBERY when one was found to have a knife and one stole a phone. Neither was him but 'joint enterprise' meant he was still arrested.

- Eighteen-year-old boy ARRESTED FOR FRAUD for caring too much, wanting to help people and bending a rule.

All these teens managed to escape these arrests unscathed because they had strong, caring parents who stood by them and fought for the ADHD to be recognised as the protagonist in all these situations. A lot won't be as blessed with parents like this so you may well find yourself the main source of support if a student of yours lands up in trouble.

If the child is lucky enough to have supportive parents and they are involved, there is a lot of information here that is hopefully going to help but firstly – tell them there is no need to PANIC nor CRY! It is incredibly common for ADHD kids to get into trouble with the law. So they ARE NOT ALONE. Dozens of parents of ADHD kids are entering this nightmare every day of the week, all over the world. There are numerous reasons for this. ADHD kids get a real thrill/buzz/adrenaline shot from stealing things. And that's just for starters.

I've mentioned earlier that I used to steal as a twelve- to thirteen-year-old. And I became extremely adept at it! Every Friday my mother would pull up outside the newsagents and I would go in to collect the family comics and magazines, which were a weekly treat. It was a very old newsagents with all the sweets laid out in rows between me and the shopkeeper. As he turned his back to get the magazines, I hastily and swiftly filled my pockets with chocolate bars and sweets. I did this for quite a few months.

I can't begin to tell you the absolute buzz I got from doing this. It is still probably the most thrilling thing I have ever done. I wasn't frightened of the shopkeeper catching me: I was confident I could predict his turning round in time to stop. But I was scared my spoils would fall out of the heavily slanted, shallow pockets of my navy-blue school raincoat in the car. I was more terrified of my mother's reaction to my thieving than of any shopkeeper!

I can still remember the extreme adrenaline rush this gave me, which is perhaps why I understand the tens of thousands of ADHD young offenders in prison for doing pretty much the same thing. So, firstly, understand that whatever the child is up to is probably giving them a massive dose of adrenaline.

It might not be stealing, although that is the number one reason ADHD kids first get into trouble with the law. Also up there at the top of the list is criminal damage because they do like to kick, especially when they're having a meltdown. Other highly probables are assault, fighting and drugs. All of these will be giving the child a thrill, which their brain will be absolutely loving and wanting more of.

Next, we need to take into account the ADHD traits of risk-taking, thrill-seeking, pushing boundaries and having no respect for authority. You don't need me to explain why those push ADHD kids into doing naughty stuff. The threat of parents, teachers or police pale into insignificance compared to the incredible thrill and excitement these bring.

Boredom comes into play here, too. I've lost count of the ADHD young offenders I've worked with who say they committed their crimes because they were bored and there was nothing else to do. Add into these traits the fact that ADHD kids are often restless, wanting to get out and DO something. That 'do something' can easily turn into something risky. Quite simply because anything boring doesn't appeal to their brain.

Another huge factor is that an ADHD brain doesn't have the ability to think of the consequence. It will think of the initial excitement without thinking of the consequence for one second.

Medication should help greatly so, if the child is not yet on ADHD medication, or (as is common) has stopped taking it at the point of getting into trouble with the law, urge the parents to reconsider getting the child on medication, pronto. This should reduce the risk-taking and thrill-seeking urges and should also allow the child to think of the consequences of their actions, which they just won't do without ADHD-specific medication.

There are two scenarios I'm now going to talk you through. One is where the police are already involved, and the other is where they aren't. Let's start with when they aren't.

If you manage to catch the child doing something illegal and the police are not involved, that is the time to take very swift and positive action. If the parents have the funds, encourage them to book the child straight in with an ADHD coach, one who understands fully the impact their behaviour is going to have on their life. Be careful if you have a school counsellor. If they don't have ADHD themselves OR a huge understanding of it and ALL the traits, they can do more damage than good. That's not a sweeping statement. If the school counsellor doesn't understand how an ADHD brain works they just aren't going to understand the student's way of thinking. And strategies and techniques that work for neurotypical kids won't touch the sides when it comes to an ADHD brain.

The most crucial bit of advice I can give you and their parents is that you must let the child know you are ON THEIR SIDE. If you take up an oppositional stance, things are definitely going to get worse. And potentially a lot worse. The more distance you create in your relationship, the more the child is going to enjoy shocking and annoying you with their behaviour.

I always suggest whichever parent is communicating best with the child at this time (if you have the choice of two), get THEM to have a very quiet but serious conversation away from everyone else. It is imperative that they let the child know they are ON THEIR SIDE. They need to know that as long as they are being honest with parents and supportive teachers, you've all got their back and will do everything in your power to get them out of the current situation.

They won't show it but I can guarantee that child will be terrified. They will cover it up with all sorts of arrogance and bolshiness but trust me: inside, each of them will be absolutely terrified and feeling very out of control. So ignore whatever abuse they throw at you and remember inside they are a frightened child.

Next, they need to appreciate the severity of the situation. Without scaring them and without telling them off, you need to help them understand the impact of what they have done. Remember, their brain won't automatically have thought of the consequences so you need to explain what the worst-case scenarios could be, at the same time assuring them of your absolute commitment to helping them get out of this situation.

These consequences could be having a criminal record, limited career options and reduced travel opportunities. A top tip: the ADHD child could have thought about going to prison, but they won't have thought that they might not be able to go to America. Do your fact-finding about their particular criminal activity and what could be the long-term consequences.

When you talk to them about these consequences it is very important you do it from a positive angle. For example, 'Thank goodness we've caught this early, and if you change your behaviour now these things won't affect you.' Always keep it positive. Everything you say can be presented in a positive light; remember, how you interact with an ADHD brain is very indicative of the response you will get.

Once they have understood you are all on their side, make it very clear that they have to be brutally honest with you about everything they have done in the past, so you are fully aware of what you are dealing with.

Also make it clear that you understand blips may happen again in the near future and the ONLY THING you ask of them is that they are honest with you. Reiterate how you will not judge; you understand that ADHD drives them to do certain things but if you are to get them out of this situation, they HAVE to be absolutely honest with you, to give you the best chance of helping them.

At this point you need to let them know that blips are part and parcel of life. Nobody is ever going to be 100% perfect and with ADHD they are prone to making more mistakes than other people, especially as they are growing up and entering the adult world. There are going to be lots of opportunities to screw things up. However, the more aware they are of how their brain operates, and the more honest they are with you, the more you can all keep blips to an absolute minimum.

I can't stress enough the importance of letting them know there will always be blips. My work with offenders in prisons proved this.

When I was trying to get the naughtiest of boys to change their behaviour, once they had accepted that a blip didn't mean a failure and also didn't mean they weren't changing their behaviour long-term, they were honest with me when one happened and we used each of them as a learning opportunity. I can still remember their little faces as I walked into the room. Before I'd sat down they'd be telling me of their blip – so desperate were they to be honest.

I never chastised, always congratulated them for being honest and then we dissected what had happened and put in place how they wanted to handle it next time. We used every single blip as a learning opportunity. What worked, what didn't. What might have made a difference. This works just as well for kids on the outside!

Analysing their actions makes them pay attention to what they inattentively did before without thinking of the consequence. Pure ADHD. You can help them see things differently. The very fact that you tell them you know there will be blips, guarantees there will be a lot less of them, in my experience.

Remember, ADHD brains are reward based at this point. So a whole list of negatives is not going to help you. What is going to help you is telling the child any of the following that is relevant:

- By being honest and changing behaviours now, they are giving themselves the best chance of keeping all their options open when they get to sixteen/eighteen/twenty-one.

- By being honest and owning up to their mistakes now, they can avoid having a criminal record.

- Having no criminal record means they can go in the forces if they choose to. They won't be restricted in any of their career choices.

- Changing their behaviour now means they won't be restricted as to which countries they can travel to (and restrictions often last for the rest of their life).

- Remind them that ADHD people do not like being told what to do. Yet if they carry on with their criminal activities all those choices are going to be taken away. The police and subsequently possibly the prison and probation service will be telling them what to do, when and what to eat, when they can sleep and controlling every aspect of their day. No ADHD person wants this. Make it abundantly clear to the child that they still have ALL the choices and if they want to be in charge of their own life they just need to change their current behaviour.

- Make it very clear to them that this is THEIR choice. If they want to choose a life with no freedom and being told what to do, it is absolutely their choice to carry on their illegal activities. But if they want to be in charge of their own life, they need to work with you to change what they are doing – and quick. Remember, ADHD people do not like being told what to do, so you have to make it very clear that all the choices are in their hands.

If you take this approach you have the strongest chance of the ADHD child changing their behaviour. This works in about 90% of cases. The other 10% are kids who are hellbent on a criminal lifestyle and with those you've really got your work cut out. Often these kids have relatives in prison telling them how it's not that bad inside and that they shouldn't worry about doing a bit of low-level crime as a short spell in prison won't do them any harm and is worth it! Or they have older friends who have been in prison and come out telling whopping great lies about their time inside – actually to protect their own status – but this leads to younger kids thinking it's cool to be a gangster or a dealer or a robber. It's really not. There is nothing cool about being locked up in a cell twenty-three hours a day and treated like dirt, which is all the prison service has lined up for them.

For these exceptionally strong-willed, bullish characters you may well need to bring in outside help. There are organisations who specifically work with kids like this. My own, Headstuff ADHD Liberty, offers highly specific counselling and coaching to keep ADHD kids away from a criminal lifestyle.

But please don't you give up, even with the most difficult, hard-to-reach teenagers. You need to be consistent, positive, always on their side and gently pushing for them to make the right choices. It is probable that at some point they will realise what you are saying makes sense. Expect them to fight you every step of the way but do not give up!

You'll need incredible resilience, and it is always wise for parents to call in help from other members of the family who can communicate most easily with the child. Often, this could be an auntie, uncle, or grandparent. I've worked with the most prolific offenders for years who suddenly have that lightbulb moment and realise what I'm saying makes sense. So don't give up. You could be in this for the long haul.

Now for the alternative scenario, when the police are already involved. All of the above still applies but in addition I strongly recommend you advise the parents to find a solicitor who understands ADHD. They do exist, and as time goes by, more and more of them are becoming aware of the condition and its link with criminal behaviour.

Since I left the prison service, I've been working in private practice specialising in helping ADHD teens and young adults who are finding themselves on the wrong side of the law. After a lot of research, investigating countless recommendations and sitting through actual court proceedings, and by a ruthless process of elimination, I have managed to find some of the best ADHD solicitors and barristers in the country. Get in touch with me and I can link you up with them.

My strong advice to the parents would be to not entertain engaging a solicitor who doesn't have extensive experience with ADHD. If the child also has a diagnosis of ASD it is even more important that the solicitor has knowledge of both conditions.

Don't just assume a local highly reputable solicitor is going to know enough about neurodiversity to represent an ADHD child. I've seen parents go this route and it has always gone horribly wrong. Just having a good solicitor isn't good enough when you are dealing with ADHD. They need to know about all the different ADHD traits, how they have impacted on the child, their connection to crime generally and this particular crime specifically. Ideally, enlist the help of an

ADHD coach to instruct your legal team on the different ADHD traits that will have contributed to the crime.

It is not a given, but in every court case I've been involved in, as long as the solicitor has a thorough understanding of ADHD, the diagnosis has been enough to keep the ADHD child out of prison. Should this child not yet have been diagnosed, or medicated, or on the right dose of the right medication, these factors also play a huge part in the judge's decision, go in the child's favour and count as mitigating evidence.

Make sure the parents are keeping a list of the important dates, diagnosis, dose of what medication they were on and for how long and all communication between themselves and their GP and ADHD psychiatrist. This can become critical in court.

It can be a hugely scary time for families when ADHD teenagers get into trouble with the law. A supportive teacher, who knows what the child and their parents are going through, will change the child's life at school. Accept that their fear and uncertainty about what's happening will often make them distracted, surly and not bothered about studying because they're thinking, 'What's the point? I'll be in prison soon.' They will very possibly be aggressive, snappy, sarcastic and rude. Make allowances for this; I can almost guarantee it's coming from a place of fear and anxiety, although it may look very different!

Often, the families themselves have been very law-abiding, highly respected professional people and are horrified that a member of the family has become involved with the police. Try to keep them calm. Let them know that this is very probably happening right now to another ADHD child in another class. And most certainly in the same town. It is very, very common and with the right legal support and with the child knowing you are all completely on their side, there is a way through.

I know many families who have been distraught when the police have entered their teenage child's life but, with the right help and the right support from school, they really can navigate through this.

Colleges and universities all over the UK are full of ADHD kids who nearly screwed it up completely, but turned it round. Look at some of the best ADHD examples out there. Sir Richard Branson went to prison at twenty for tax evasion. It is totally possible to change the child's life path, with your support.

TOP TEACHING TIPS … Don't go into a massive panic. This has happened before, and it will happen again, with ADHD children. Don't feel like their world has ended and this is catastrophic for them. It's not. It's due to their ADHD and it's common.

There is professional help at hand and the parents will gain much-needed support having an understanding teacher working with their child at school. Don't take the oppositional stance with the child. Don't chastise them and make them feel worse than they probably already do, even if they are playing the big 'I am' and 'I don't care' to your face.

WHAT WORKS BEST … Keep the lines of communication open. Let the child know you are on their side. Assure them that you will get through this together. Accept that they might be more stroppy and aggressive than usual but this is almost definitely covering up fear and anxiety inside.

Work with the parents and advise them to seek help and always deal with legal professionals who fully understand ADHD.

Important stuff I want to remember:

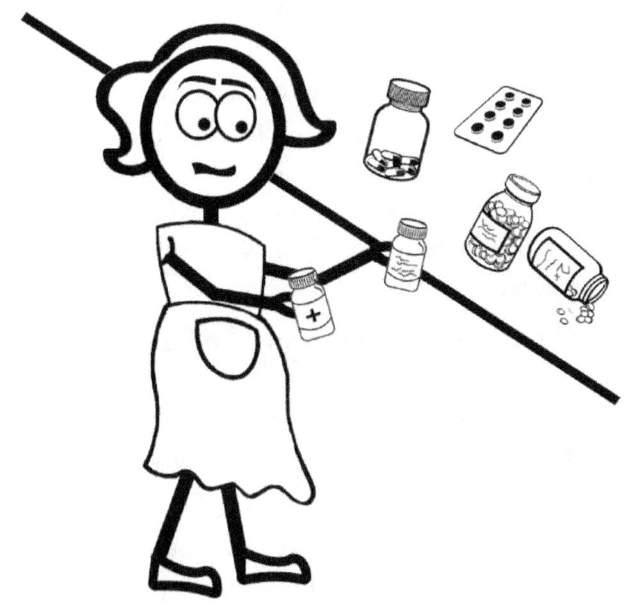

WHAT YOU NEED TO KNOW ABOUT ADHD MEDICATION

Before starting this section I'm going to make it extremely clear that I am in no way medically qualified. I am not a GP, psychiatrist or psychologist. I am but a humble counsellor who has worked with hundreds of ADHD clients. What I'm about to tell you has been gleaned from my experience working with parents who do or don't give their children medication, and the children and adolescents taking it. It is their experiences that I will be using, hopefully to give you a better understanding of what ADHD medication can do for an ADHD child.

As a teacher you might be surprised to find that parents may well ask you for your opinion on whether to medicate their child or not. The reason for this is that it is often a child's education that is affected most by them not being medicated. So the parents could well base their decision on whether to medicate or not on your opinion. For that reason, it will be more than handy for you to understand what ADHD meds can do for a child, and also the most common side-effects as well as how taking medication will affect them at school.

Usually when a child is first diagnosed ADHD the parents will be given the option of medication. Paediatricians and psychiatrists typically leave the decision of whether to medicate or not up to Mum or Dad and the vast majority of parents find this scary and unhelpful. They've no idea what they are supposed to do and there is hardly any information out there.

I try hard to fill that gap for them – and now for you. But please always remember this is based on my own experience and that of my clients and is NOT medical advice. For that, the parents absolutely must speak to an ADHD paediatrician or psychiatrist.

The initial reaction of most parents to being offered ADHD medication for their child is, 'Not on your life.' The thought of putting medication into their precious poppet's perfect, tiny body is the last thing they want to do. And I understand this perfectly. I really do.

ADHD medication is notoriously confusing but, trying to keep it simple, there are two main types: non-stimulant and stimulant. Stimulants nearly always work much better for ADHD, but for people who can't tolerate the stimulants then the non-stimulants are an alternative. Stimulant names that you will hear bandied about are Elvanse, Concerta and Dexamphetamine. Non-stimulants are Atomoxetine, also known as Strattera, and Guanfacine.

Knowing what I know now, I think NOT trying medication is nearly always the wrong decision. And I don't say that lightly.

Because by not giving an ADHD child medication what you are in actual fact doing is forcing their brain to work 24/7 in the way it doesn't want to. The child will be having to force their brain to focus, to concentrate, to sit still, not fiddle, not get bored, not be distracted, not say and do things impulsively without thinking of the consequence, not joke, not be the clown of the class. Because that's what it WANTS to do and by not medicating we are going to be asking them to NOT do that without any assistance whatsoever!

Not medicating is also not giving the child the best chance at their education, because the medication helps them concentrate and focus. Crucially, medication also helps them retain information. Remember, an ADHD brain rarely thinks a thought long enough for it to be stored as a memory. How difficult is it going to make revision for the child if they don't have the benefit of medication helping them retain their thoughts?

And this isn't just going to affect them at school. Think about them going on to college and perhaps even university. Asking their brain to override itself through all those years is going to be taxing and they will pay a price.

ADHD children who aren't medicated are the ones who usually wing it at GCSEs, invariably fail at A-level when they have to focus on fewer subjects, and if they manage to get through A levels they nearly always crash at university because the stress and pressure of behaving in a way that your brain doesn't want to will always impact them in the end. There's a lot of other reasons why ADHD kids struggle when it comes to university but, trust me, the ones on medication have a much better chance of making it.

There are tons of other very good reasons why it is sensible to at least try medication.

If the ADHD child is one who suffers with emotional dysregulation or anxiety, the medication, when it is working, can have a hugely positive effect. I would go so far as to say it can completely eradicate unstable moods and therefore lessen the likelihood of self-harm and suicidal thoughts. Unregulated ADHD teenage emotions can be extreme, and the medication can have a life-changing positive effect on emotionally unstable teenagers.

And there are more positive benefits of medication.

- Meds can motivate the child. Without even noticing it, the child will have a lot more motivation to do things, including the boring things!

- Meds should pretty much stop procrastination so homework, tidying up, hygiene and other tasks that have been put off before will suddenly start getting done.

- Meds will allow the child to think a thought for long enough for it to be stored as a memory. So things that up to now have regularly been forgotten, like lunchboxes and PE kits, should suddenly be remembered.

- Meds should also stop, or at least dramatically reduce, impulsivity. An ADHD child is less likely to lose friends and they will upset fewer teachers because they won't be saying and doing things without thinking.

- The child on meds should now be able to think of consequences. I can't begin to tell you how important this one is. If I tell you that most of the prisons are full of ADHD boys who didn't think of the consequence before committing silly crimes, you'll know that putting this ability back into an ADHD child's brain is critical and could very well be life-altering.

Have I convinced you that trying medication is a good idea yet? If not, I'll keep going!

If the child has had any sort of binge-eating problem, or uncontrolled eating, compulsively eating sweets, stealing or gorging on food, the medication will regulate their appetite and stop compulsivity in its tracks. Even the non-stimulants do this.

Medication should also calm their brain and stop the racing thoughts. Most ADHD kids have brains that don't stop, and the medication will actually allow them to think one thought from the beginning to the end. This is a completely novel idea for anybody with ADHD who has constant crashing thoughts ricocheting round their brain. A calm brain has to be one of the best things the medication brings.

I can speak personally on this. On the few occasions I've tried ADHD stimulant medication the effect in my brain has been nothing less than earth-shattering. For the first time EVER, I knew what it felt like to have a brain that was calm, that wasn't incessantly thinking and overthinking. Quite honestly it was the best thing since sliced bread and although I have my own reasons at the moment for still struggling to be on stimulant medication, it is my absolute goal to get back on it because this effect is truly wonderful.

So now we can see the medication, when it works, is pretty fantastic but there have to be side-effects right? And yes, there are. I always say to clients that ADHD medication has to be the hardest to get on BUT when you are on it and it is working it has to be the best in the world. I'm not exaggerating here because ADHD medication is known as the most efficacious of all medication – because it is the only one that replaces something missing in the brain.

But let's talk side-effects.

There aren't that many, but they can be bad enough to turn people off the meds altogether. I'll list these in the order they seem to affect the thousands of ADHD people I have now met and worked with.

SLEEP

Quite a large proportion of people find they cannot sleep on stimulant medication. I've known people who have been awake for a week when they first take it. This is obviously very dangerous, and I send all of them straight back to their psychiatrist. Some psychiatrists will give you additional sleep medication to counteract the effect of a stimulant. Melatonin is very popular with children and teens, and medication to calm your brain down at night can be very useful for adults. More than any other side-effect, I'm positive disrupted sleep has to be the top one.

LACK OF APPETITE

Now for some of us carrying a few extra pounds (who am I kidding – stones), this one isn't such a horror and it can't be a coincidence that the first-line medication for ADHD, Elvanse, is also prescribed for binge eating. Some people however find their appetite is wiped out to quite a dangerous degree. Kids can go days without eating and then only realise when they faint in school.

BAD MOOD/MELTDOWNS/ANXIETY WHEN THEY WEAR OFF

Not so much with Elvanse but other, older-style, ADHD medication can cause some people to have a terrible 'crash' late in the afternoon when it wears off. Parents report children suddenly becoming very angry, wired and emotional; this is the effect of the medication leaving their brain.

DRY MOUTH AND BEING CONSTANTLY THIRSTY

It is recommended that you drink a lot of water when you are taking ADHD medication. For some reason it makes it work better. They also recommend that you have protein in the morning and at lunchtime if you are taking Elvanse. Apparently that helps meds work better, too.

ANXIETY/CHEST PAIN/HEART PALPITATIONS

This is rare but if it does happen and the child tells you this is happening make sure you advise the parents to consult their child's paediatrician or psychiatrist immediately. They will usually tell them to stop taking the medication and make an appointment to see them. This is very unusual but if it does happen obviously it needs to be taken very seriously.

Something I come across a lot is boys in their late teens who have decided they no longer need their ADHD medication. I always meet the ones who have hit major trouble as a result. A lot of boys seem to think that they only needed the meds for school, or when they were a kid, and they are fine without them. Hardly ever is this the case.

We now know that we are born with ADHD and we die with it. It is absolutely not a childhood disorder that you grow out of in your late teens. But this old urban myth still floats around and many with ADHD also believe it is true. My therapy room is chock-a-block with seventeen to nineteen-year-olds thinking they don't need the medication anymore and not yet linking their dismissal of meds to the fact their lives have gone very wrong.

Most parents have the devil's own job talking these headstrong teenagers back into taking medication. I have tried too and the best way I've found is to tell them they only need to try it in the short term, for a week or two, and see if it makes a difference. If it doesn't, they can just stop taking it. There is no long-term build-up with ADHD medication so you literally can take it for a week or a fortnight and then stop with no negative impacts. Hopefully in this time they will have seen the difference being back on meds can make.

Medication isn't right for everybody, of course, but from what I've seen, it has a dramatically positive effect on most people with ADHD. Encourage ADHD kids not to give up at the first hurdle. They might need to try two, or even more, different kinds of medication to find the right fit but, generally speaking, the positive effects are numerous and worth persevering for.

TOP TEACHING TIPS … Be prepared to answer parents' questions about whether their child's ADHD is impacting their concentration, their focus, their ability to learn, their ability to keep friendships and not be impulsive and distracted. Be aware that when a child is starting or changing medication it may affect their moods and attitude quite dramatically.

WHAT WORKS BEST … Watch and monitor how the ADHD child is coping, especially around temper, meltdowns, concentrating, focusing and emotionally. If you know a child is medicated and their abilities seem to be lessening, have a conversation with the parents about whether a medication review might be wise to help with their education.

Understand that medication wearing off in the early afternoon often means children are less able to concentrate and focus and will be more fidgety, hyperactive and restless as the afternoon goes on. So if yours is a school with later lessons or after-school classes and activities, expect to see a change in the ADHD child who is medicated.

Important stuff I want to remember:

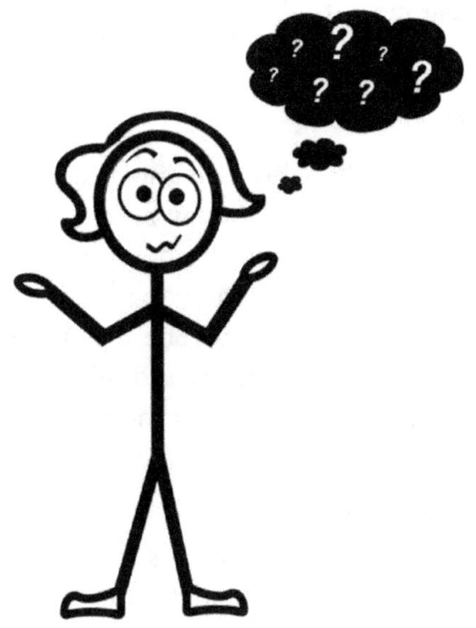

WHEN YOU ARE ASKED FOR YOUR OPINION ON THERAPY

The good news is there is now quite a lot of choice when it comes to professional help you can access for ADHD children. The sad news is that, in the UK at least, most of this isn't available on the NHS or for free and parents will need to access the help privately. But if they can afford it, then the ADHD-specific help is there.

Some schools have budgets to refer children for private therapy and on rare occasions it does happen. Social Services will fund ADHD-specific therapy for a child especially when the parents can't afford it and the child is considered to be at risk in some way – usually with offending behaviour.

There are charitable organisations who offer therapeutic services for ADHD kids and their parents and in the 'Where to Find More ADHD Support' section at the back of the book you will find details on some of those.

Sometimes it can be very obvious an ADHD child needs additional support and some sort of therapeutic intervention but it's not so easy to fathom just what the right sort of help is. It can be a confusing quagmire of job titles but I'll try to make sense of them for you.

ADHD COACH

This is somebody who is almost definitely not a qualified counsellor. If they were, they would mention it in their job title. An ADHD coach is likely to be somebody who has taken a specific coaching course on everything ADHD. Most of these at the moment are USA-based. These coaches will be able to help the parents and child understand all the ADHD traits they are dealing with and come up with the best tried-and-tested coping strategies and techniques to overcome these issues.

What they won't be able to do is deal with emotions and feelings to the depth a counsellor can. They won't be trained in areas such as self-harm, suicidal ideation, self-esteem, body dysmorphia, eating disorders, anger management, anxiety, depression and a whole catalogue of other issues. A counsellor will.

There are some very professional ADHD coaches available and they most certainly have their place. In my personal opinion, that place is working with adults who have no other issues aside from their ADHD traits. Mostly, children will have other issues which will be best dealt with by a qualified counsellor.

ADHD COUNSELLOR/PSYCHOTHERAPIST

These people will have undertaken a minimum of three years – probably more like four or five years – training in counselling and psychotherapy, often to degree and master's level. Somewhere along the line they will also have gained ADHD knowledge. This is nearly always because they have ADHD themselves and have chosen to specialise in this area. You will also find parents of ADHD children who are qualified counsellors, offering ADHD counselling services.

My advice here would be to always look at the therapist's own website rather than a national counselling database. On these you'll see they have ticked ADHD as a client group they work with. In reality, this could mean they have worked with one or two ADHD children before and won't turn away clients with

ADHD. It doesn't mean they specialise in ADHD or even know much about it. Counsellors tend to tick all these boxes in the hope they will attract more clients.

In my view, a child or adolescent is going to need a counsellor, not a coach. I think coaches are ideal when there are no emotional or additional issues but I've yet to meet a child with ADHD who isn't also suffering with low self-esteem, health anxiety, depression, eating issues, bullying, friendship group problems, self-harm or any one of another hundred issues.

I qualified as a coach before I trained as a counsellor. In our coaching training we were told that if a client presents with emotional issues we had to refer them to a counsellor. Now I am trained as a counsellor I can completely see why this is the case. There is absolutely no point in working with a child on just their ADHD traits if there are underlying issues – and there nearly always are with ADHD.

Let's think first of the 30% of ADHD kids who have social anxiety. In counselling there are a lot of ways of working with anxiety, for example CBT is known to be extremely successful. An ADHD coach will not have been trained in getting to the root of the client's anxiety, let alone know how to deal with it.

So think very carefully whether a child just needs help purely with ADHD traits. If they do then an ADHD coach will be sufficient. But if there is anything else going on like anxiety, depression, problems with siblings, self-harm etc, it is much better they are seen by a counsellor who specialises in ADHD. And for that you ideally need a counsellor who is diagnosed ADHD themselves. Nobody will understand an ADHD child's brain like somebody with the same brain themselves.

It is why my organisations, Headstuff ADHD Therapy and Headstuff ADHD Liberty, will only supply counsellors who have an ADHD diagnosis to work with ADHD clients. What we hear from clients over and over again is that it is amazing sitting in front of somebody who understands their brain.

You will now find people who are qualified counsellors AND coaches. I am one of these. Until a few years ago that was pretty rare. Now it is becoming more common as the UK embraces coaching, and counsellors are following up their training with coaching training.

I did it the other way around and became a coach ten years before I became a counsellor. But you will find combined ADHD coaches and counsellors now, and personally I think that's the best option. The choices are out there for parents to make but don't undervalue your own input as their teacher. You will be seeing their child interacting with others for six or seven hours a day. You are much more likely to pick up whether they have friendship issues, social anxiety, emotional dysregulation, rejection sensitivity and other issues that can be dealt with very well in therapy.

CBT THERAPIST

This will be a professional who has undertaken specific CBT training. If they don't have ADHD themselves, or a massive understanding of it, they aren't going to be much use to an ADHD child. But a counsellor trained in CBT who is ADHD themselves is definitely worth considering. We have them on our team and they are fabulous at working with clients when their thinking is the cause of most of their problems. Overthinking, busy brain, rumination, rejection sensitive dysphoria, emotional dysregulation are all ADHD traits and all 'thinking problems' – and CBT deals with identifying negative thoughts and changing thought patterns.

ADHD PSYCHOLOGIST/PSYCHIATRIST

These top-layer people will only usually sit in front of the child and their parents when they are first looking for an assessment for ADHD or medication for the condition. Psychologists can diagnose the condition, but only psychiatrists can medicate as well as diagnose. Neither usually offer any form of psychotherapy. Sometimes psychologists do but most lack the counselling skills to work long-term with clients.

It is also worth mentioning at this point that in the UK a GP cannot initiate the prescription of ADHD medication. That has to come from a consultant at psychiatrist level. This is because (most) ADHD medications are controlled so a regular GP can dispense prescriptions but cannot initiate a prescription for them.

SCHOOL COUNSELLOR

This might be the only option you can offer parents but please tread extremely carefully. If you are referring a student to the school counsellor, and you know the child has ADHD, do make sure the therapist knows this. As I write, ADHD does not feature in counselling training so there is no guarantee your school counsellor will have been made aware of how ADHD people think differently.

You might strike gold and find that your school counsellor has their own ADHD diagnosis. I know this happens because some of our Headstuff therapists work in schools! So you are onto a winner in that scenario.

But if the therapist knows nothing about ADHD, and the school counsellor really is the only option because parents can't afford to pay privately, do make sure at the very least the therapist reads up on ADHD before working with the client, or ideally does some continuing professional development training on ADHD.

Important stuff I want to remember:

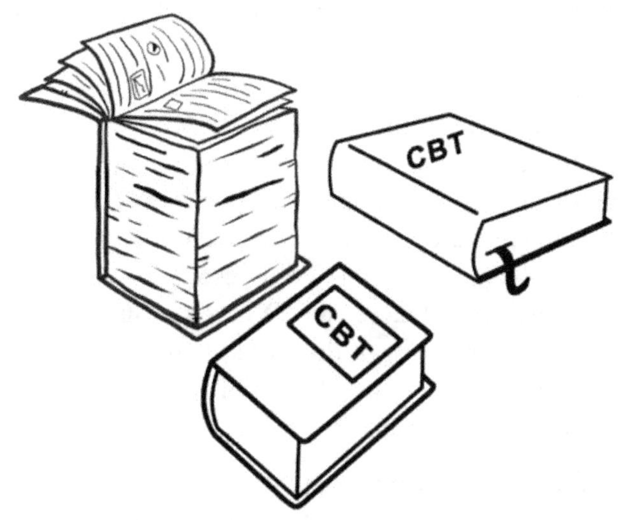

SOME BASIC CBT SKILLS

CBT stands for Cognitive Behavioural Therapy and you hear the term bandied about so much because the NHS in the UK has been using it as the preferred choice of therapy for a good few years. The reason they use it so much is because, more than any other counselling method, CBT is evidence based: you go from A to B and you get a result. The NHS want to be able to evidence results.

So what is it all about and can it help your ADHD students – in fact ALL your students? My answer to that is a definite YES. If your school has emotional literacy or emotional intelligence lessons, CBT could fit very nicely there. In the UK schools include 'personal, social, health and economic education' and the basics of CBT most definitely are very useful in the health element, particularly relating to mental health.

I'm going to go through the relevant areas of CBT here, very much picking out the elements I think work brilliantly with ADHD kids. However there is no reason why this won't be helpful for ALL students and it will certainly make them all more aware of how their thoughts affect their feelings, which in turn affect their behaviour.

I've literally seen CBT work, and help, dozens and dozens of times. And it is simple enough for even a ten-year-old to grasp the basics.

If you want to go into CBT more thoroughly, I can strongly recommend three excellent websites. These have tons of information, CBT exercises and even full CBT programmes that you can download. The programmes each specialise in one problem area. Examples are self-esteem, body dysmorphia, health anxiety, procrastination, worry and rumination, and there are loads of them. Each programme has around ten to twelve modules and if any child has one real problem area, this is a free resource which will almost definitely be very powerful. See the 'Where to Find More ADHD Support' section at the back of this book. I suspect some of them (the self-esteem one, for example) would be very useful to do as class projects. They are a great free resource for teachers.

However, if it is general CBT you'd like to get a handle on to help all your students but particularly those overthinking, ruminating, busy-brain ADHD ones, keep reading!

Broken down, CBT means 'cognitive' (your brain and how you think), 'behaviour' (how you behave) 'therapy' (changing for the better). So its basis is changing your thoughts to change your feelings and behaviour for the better. There's not a child in the world who won't benefit from understanding that.

You might have heard of the CBT hot cross bun. Before you reach for the butter and start salivating it is actually a diagram of THOUGHTS, FEELINGS, BEHAVIOURS, PHYSICAL SYMPTOMS and how one leads on to the others (not necessarily in any set order).

The theory is that whatever the problem, you can break the circle at any point to change the end result. Let's take an easy example. If a child is depressed, their thoughts, when identified, might be 'I'm boring, nobody likes me, I've got no friends'. This might leave them feeling sad, lonely and rejected, which might lead to them isolating themselves, not going out, not answering the phone and staying in bed. Their physical sensations may be feeling sick and tired.

To break the cycle, a CBT therapist will enter the hot cross bun at the point where it can have the most effect AND where it is most do-able for the client. In this case I would suggest a behavioural change might have instant impact. Starting by answering the telephone and going out once a week. Baby steps. This is the core of CBT therapy.

The area that I think is most helpful to both ADHD and neurotypical kids is around UNHELPFUL THINKING STYLES. This is massively relevant. Two of the biggest traits of ADHD are overthinking and ruminating. I've yet to meet one ADHD person who doesn't overthink to a lesser or greater degree. Many tell me it is their worst trait and the one that gives them the most grief. I believe it is responsible for nearly all the anxiety we suffer and can be life-threatening in its extreme. People who self-harm will always tell you it was their thoughts they were trying to escape from.

Some thoughts are positive. In CBT these are called 'positive automatic thoughts' (PATs). And the opposite of these are 'negative automatic thoughts' (NATs). These are the ones all children will need help recognising and changing. And that's not as hard as you think. I recommend you have a look at the ten most common unhelpful thinking styles. How many apply to you? This is a great place to start with kids.

BLACK-AND-WHITE THINKING

Also known as All-or-Nothing Thinking. This is classic ADHD. For us, everything is either brilliant or it is absolutely awful. Try getting children to look at grey areas instead. Are there any? How many different ways can they look at things?

CATASTROPHISING

Always assuming the very worst. Again, classic ADHD! Nothing is ever just a bit rubbish; for us it is always a total disaster! Instead, encourage children to keep it real. What do they know? What are all the possible outcomes, not just the worst?

EMOTIONAL REASONING

Assuming that because something makes you feel a certain way it must be true. For example, 'I feel stupid in maths so I must be thick'. Instead, encourage, 'I don't feel confident yet in maths so maybe I'd benefit from one-to-one sessions with a teacher or a private tutor'.

LABELLING

Making global statements or assumptions about ourselves to others for example, 'Everyone in my class is horrid because they all hate me'. Instead, think who has ever been kind to me, or helped me? Do they all deserve to be labelled?

MAGNIFICATION AND MINIMISATION

Building other people up, putting them on pedestals, and belittling yourself or your own attributes, achievements and skills. This feeds in beautifully with ADHD's lack of self-esteem! Remind your students they only see what other people want them to see. Very often people present completely differently publicly. Instead, focus on themselves and know their own worth. There is no point second-guessing other people.

MENTAL FILTER

Not seeing the full picture. Filtering out the good bits and only registering the bad. Again, classic ADHD automatic thoughts. Instead, explore what they might have missed.

MIND-READING AND FORTUNE-TELLING

Thinking we know what someone is thinking or how something is going to pan out. Instead, ask children to stay in the now. Encourage their brain to think only of what they have evidence for. Some basic mindfulness comes in very handy for this.

OVER-GENERALISING

Imagining something always happens, based solely on one event. Typical ADHD; we can be dramatic! Instead, check out the evidence. How many times has it actually happened?

PERSONALISATION

Taking everything personally. Always thinking you are responsible and everything is your fault. Instead, try looking around. Who else is involved? What part might other people have played in this?

'SHOULD' AND 'MUST' THINKING

Being hard on yourself by using phrases like 'I should', 'I must', 'I ought to'. Rarely is this thinking helpful. Instead, help children replace these phrases with 'it would be nice if', 'I might' and 'I could'.

HOT TIP! This CBT-based statement I have found to be the most powerful one ever:

A THOUGHT IS JUST A THOUGHT. IT IS NOT NECESSARILY A FACT.

Think about it for a minute. This is crucially important for ADHD brains as we have more thoughts than most and a good portion of those are negative. But they are just thoughts. That does not mean they are true or factual.

If you can just get this bit of CBT into an ADHD child's head, you'll help them so much. An ADHD brain can fire off hundreds of thoughts in a day and if you can help the child to understand that a thought really is just a thought, it will do wonders for their mental health.

I'm a very big believer in CBT and there are hundreds of books on the subject. There are specifically books for using CBT with children and adolescents so if you want to go further into this, I strongly recommend it. For me it is by far and away the best counselling method to work with ADHD brains. And it won't hurt your other students to understand it too. ADHD kids aren't the only ones with low self-esteem and thoughts that run away with themselves.

Important stuff I want to remember:

SOME 'AT HOME' SITUATIONS WHICH MIGHT CROSS OVER INTO SCHOOL

These next few chapters are taken from the book I wrote specifically to help parents. If you happen to be not only a teacher but also a parent of ADHD kids, you will hopefully find this information useful, which is why I have included them here.

Even if you are not a parent of an ADHD child, I still think it's helpful for you to read these few chapters to see how parents will be managing these aspects of their ADHD children's lives at home.

You can then hopefully reinforce the same strategies and techniques when they are in school.

I will explain more as we go along.

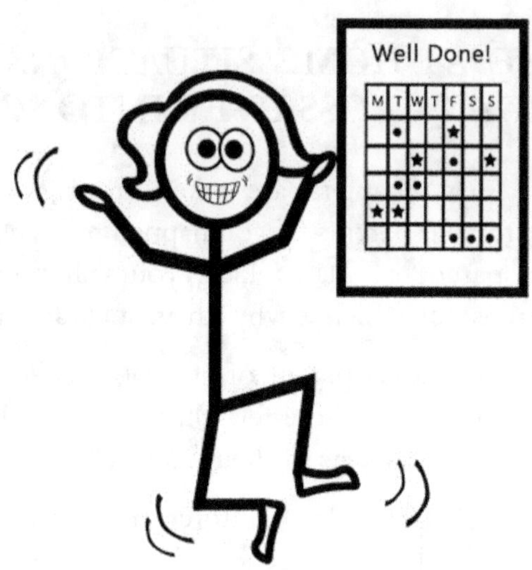

REWARD SYSTEMS

This chapter on reward systems is massively important for parents. ADHD brains are reward based so I always encourage parents to have reward systems that suit each individual ADHD child. I completely appreciate at school this might be difficult, however there will be occasions where even the smallest reward, like going out to break early, will motivate an ADHD child's brain.

But if in your school there are opportunities for even better reward systems, it's well worth you reading on as to why rewards work so well with ADHD children – as well as ADHD adults! Reward systems could literally change your life; they are the secret weapon you can use time and time again to make situations easier in the classroom. First of all, lets have a quick refresher on what's going on in an ADHD kid's brain …

ADHD brains are under-stimulated. They need excitement, adrenaline or a reward to get them to engage. If it is not exciting or doesn't involve food or pleasure, a child's ADHD brain is just not going to be very interested. However, there is one very simple way of getting their brain to show interest. And that is by giving it something it WANTS. Something exciting. Something that will give it adrenaline! And this is where reward systems come in.

Reward systems don't need to be used just ad hoc. They can be used in every area of an ADHD kid's life. The child's brain is like this 24/7 and the way to get their brain motivated is most definitely by rewarding it. I cannot stress this enough. It is not the child being wilfully difficult and not wanting to do boring things – it is their ADHD brain. Once you get this into your head and understand the importance of working with an ADHD child's brain rather than against it, life is going to be a whole lot easier.

Reward systems can range from the intricate and grandiose to the incredibly simple. A simple example would be exactly what I'm doing now. I'm writing this chapter before telling myself I can have anything to eat. I'm in my fifties and still use my own reward systems to get myself to do things. I can do that because I understand how my brain works and I can set up my own reward systems. I do it all the time. Probably every day. It is the way I get things done.

But a young child isn't going to realise this is how their brain works, so YOU are going to need to put the reward systems in place. If you haven't used reward systems before then I strongly recommend you sit down and have a really good think about what it is that excites this child. I'm going to guess it is some of these things:

At Home

- more time on the Xbox/PlayStation

- going to bed slightly later

- not having to do the washing up or empty the dishwasher or any other chore that bores them

- having the iPad for an extra half hour in the evening

- extra money to buy clothes or trainers

- tickets to see their favourite football team or band

- choosing which takeaway the family have on a Saturday night

- extra pocket money

- having friends round for a sleepover

- choosing a theme park day out

- choosing which food goes into a picnic

- picking which ice cream flavours get bought this month

- the chance to go to TGI Fridays or Nando's

At School

- being first in the lunch queue

- having longer break times

- being put in charge of picking teams

- writing answers on black/whiteboards

- being the Quiz Master

- choosing subjects & topics

Before you think about putting any reward system in place, first of all spend a good couple of weeks thinking of ALL the things that motivate and excite this child. It really doesn't matter what it is. But you'll be able to identify these things because they will be the things that this particular child will have never given you any grief over!

Another simple example is beans on toast. I loved beans on toast as a child but didn't have it very often. For me it was a massive treat. I also loved it when we had what I called a 'buffet tea'. Something where I could pick lots of bits. Both of these things would've been enough to get me motivated enough to do something boring beforehand. So think hard here; the more you come up with, the more successful you'll be.

And, teachers, it's going to be even more of a challenge for you! Are there any ways you can reward an ADHD child within school that isn't going to be seen as unfair to other children, that won't cost the school money and is 'allowed'?

The next step is identifying areas where you want the child's behaviour to change. I don't have to give you examples of this. I'm quite sure you know exactly what it is you struggle with getting the child to do. From homework to brushing their teeth to tidying their room … Your list could be quite extensive! For teachers this could be keeping their desk or locker tidy, putting their coat on the right hook or keeping their PE kit in their PE bag and not strewn across the changing room.

So next we have to put the reward system in place. There are some golden rules with reward systems, so before we start you need to have a good grasp of them.

- The reward system has to be maintained. Don't ever start something you can't keep going. For example, don't promise football tickets every month if it is going to bankrupt you. Or, at school, don't promise that a child can be first in the lunch queue if the dinner monitor is having none of that!

- It has to be clearly communicated to everybody involved. For example, it is no good Mum knowing the system and their dad not. At school, ideally all teachers who come into contact with the child should be aware of the scheme, even if they aren't participating in it. Everybody needs to be completely up to speed on what the expectations are and what the rewards are, especially if Mum lives in one house and Dad in another, or if the child has more than one teacher.

- There must be short-term goals and long-term goals. An ADHD child is going to get bored if there is no reward within a week. And a week is the ABSOLUTE MAXIMUM you should push it without them getting some sort of recompense.

- The expectations and rewards need to be visual. Remember, an ADHD child won't be able to hold the information in their head. So at home you need to get yourself a nice big whiteboard, a blackboard or some vibrant coloured pens and nice paper. It needs to be SEEN and it needs to be in the child's mind all the time.

  At school this almost definitely WON'T work: the one thing the ADHD kid won't want is to stand out. So you will need a more discreet way of keeping track of their progress.

- It needs to be collaborative. It is no good you deciding what the reward is going to be if the child isn't interested. You can come up with the suggestions, but they have to be agreed by the child. It is the only way it will work.

- It needs to be accumulative. So, for example, if they meet your behavioural expectations for a week there needs to be an extra reward for completing a full week. An ADHD child will soon get bored if they do something for five or seven days solid and there is no reward for maintaining that long.

- There must be enough benefit in it for you. If you get the balance wrong and it is all about rewards and you're not seeing much change in their behaviour, you are soon going to wish you hadn't bothered.

- The rewards need to be changed (or 'upgraded' as the child needs to see it), on a reasonably regular basis. As soon as their brain is finding something repetitive or routine they are going to need the rewards ramped up. As an incredibly rough guide I would say every three months or at school, once a term.

Now comes the bit where you need to make some decisions. The fact that you are putting rewards in place needs to be introduced to the child at the right time and when they're in the right mood. It is no good doing it when they are in a grump, tired, hungry or having major arguments with somebody in the house or classroom. Any suggestion of a reward system at these times is going to be met with hostility. Instead, make it a time when you and the child are communicating well; they're in a good mood, laughing or coming to you for a chat. Suggest it as AN IDEA. Don't TELL them they've got to do it. Explain in a positive way that you want to reward them when they do things well, and you'd like their help with putting a system in place so they can regularly have nice things. If you present the idea this way, no ADHD child is going to say no. Remember, their brain wants rewards.

Once you've come up with the rewards they would like to be included, now is the time to broach what you want them to change. Again, this needs very delicate handling. Don't say things like, 'Well you've got to stop doing this,' and, 'You've got to start doing that.' This will only put the kid's back up.

Instead, talk about how they 'struggle' to do certain stuff and you totally understand how boring these things can be. And how you want to make it 'easier' for them. Keep everything positive. Avoid the negatives. Definitely don't tell them off for anything they've been doing or not doing. Instead, assure them you understand this is how their wonderful ADHD brain works and you want to reward them when it does good things.

Once you have the child's acceptance and you've agreed COLLABORATIVELY what it is they are going to change to make their life easier, and what rewards are going to be put in place, you're good to go!

Remember, it doesn't all have to be very sophisticated; there can be daily extra rewards like, 'I've bought some Magnums so if you want to go and just quickly tidy your room we can have them afterwards.' Little simple things like this really do work.

Here are some examples of reward systems my clients have put in place for their young children and teenagers. These have WORKED, so variations on these could be a very good place for you to start.

Example 1

An eleven-year-old boy hated going to bed. His mum put in place a system whereby if he went to bed by 8 p.m., having had a shower and making no fuss, beside his bed would be a cookie and a glass of milk. If he did this for the five days during the week, he was allowed to choose the Saturday night movie and takeaway the family shared at the weekend.

Example 2

A twelve-year-old girl was very defiant and wouldn't do anything she was told. The mum put in place a system whereby if she didn't answer back and did as she was asked all week, each Saturday she would be given £15 to spend on clothes. If she managed the whole month of this behaviour, then she was given an extra £50 on the final weekend to spend as she wished.

Example 3

A thirteen-year-old client hated showering or bathing. The mum was at her wits end because the child really whiffed! They put in a reward system whereby if he had a shower every other day and at least a wash in between (if he couldn't be bothered to shower), he would be given £1 every day. If he managed this for a full week, he was given an additional £10 on Saturday to spend on anything he wanted.

Example 4

There was a very long list of things a fourteen-year-old client of mine wouldn't do. He fought against doing homework, showering, was swearing prolifically at his family and having physical fights with his sister. The mum put in individual reward systems for each behavioural change she wanted. It ranged from 50p a day for not swearing at all and £1 for every day he didn't fight with his sister. He liked it because he saw lots of different ways to make money. There were a lot of blips but on the whole the behaviour changed.

Example 5

A fifteen-year-old girl found it very hard to motivate herself to do anything. She was incredibly bright but really struggled to do homework and anything school related. Her mum put in place a reward system whereby she could choose whatever they watched on television between 8 p.m. and 9 p.m. as long as she had finished her homework before. If she managed this for a full week, she could have the roast of her choice on Sunday, with the movie of her choice. This girl had a particular love of roast dinners!

Hopefully reading these has given you some ideas for what might work for any ADHD child. Always remember ALL decisions have to be collaborative. It just won't work if they aren't.

I totally appreciate that rewards are going to have to be very different at school but, if you put your heads together with the parents to work out exactly what motivates this particular ADHD child, hopefully you can find something that will work as a reward during the school day, too.

TOP TEACHING TIPS … Never underestimate the power of reward systems. They could completely change how a child functions at school.

WHAT WORKS BEST … Give a lot of thought and liaise with the parents as to what it is that motivates this child and what behaviours it is you want them to change. Take time in putting reward systems in place and you will reap the benefits.

Remember, they work for the smallest of reasons. The ADHD brain is reward-driven 24/7. Use that to your advantage!

Important stuff I want to remember:

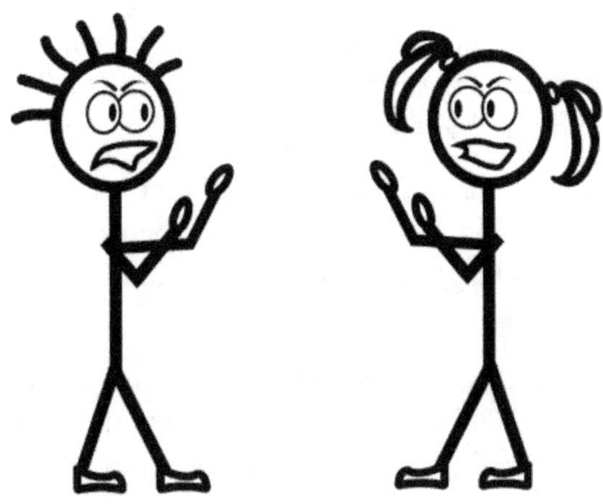

SIBLING RIVALRY

Most ADHD kids will have a variety of brothers, sisters, stepbrothers, stepsisters, half-brothers, half-sisters and some are twins or triplets. Their siblings can be older, younger or the same age. Some may live with them and some may be part-time if shared between families. And some may be at the same school. Twins might even be in the same class. We have triplets in my own family.

I've worked with hundreds of families with ADHD kids aged five to eighteen and I've seen every combination of family situation and the problems that can arise.

First, let's think about the family where there is an ADHD child and other child/ren who are neurotypical. The ADHD child is going to need special handling. This book will have told you that. So where does that leave the child without ADHD? It can leave them feeling:

- they don't get enough of their parents' attention, because all their time is taken up with the ADHD child

- that they are not special; they don't get days off for trips to the psychiatrist, medication or a 'time-out' pass at school

- that concessions are made for the ADHD child and not for them

- that they wouldn't get away with the things the ADHD child gets away with and it is not fair.

All of this can lead to resentment, hurt, anger, isolation, feelings of low self-worth and low self-esteem. And this will likely have a knock-on effect on how they feel about their sibling/s, ranging from mild dislike to full-on despising!

So my first message in this section is that it is crucially important how you treat non-ADHD siblings, for their own self-worth. They can also play a bigger part in keeping family equilibrium than you might realise.

First up, I think it is very important they know their sibling is ADHD. I have worked with families who have kept the diagnosis secret. In my view this is nearly always not the best way to handle it.[*]

Under normal circumstances I don't think it is of ANY benefit to the non-ADHD children not knowing their brother or sister has ADHD. From as early as they have understanding, I recommend you explain that they have a brother or sister whose brain works DIFFERENTLY. Not worse than theirs, and not better than theirs. But DIFFERENTLY.

It will be a lot for them to take on board. Think about how much information is in this book and then think about a young non-ADHD child taking it all in. It is an awful lot and they don't need to know everything at once. But I definitely recommend explaining a little bit more about their sibling's ADHD brain every time something happens that is ADHD related. For example, if the ADHD child:

- has a major meltdown

- is unreasonable or violent to their brother or sister

- has a serious incident at school

- gets overly emotional

- punches, kicks or attacks any family member

- gets in trouble with the police

---

[*] See the one exception at the end of this chapter.

Always have this conversation when things have calmed down (probably the next day if there has been a major issue in the house), and always in confidence. You do not want the ADHD child overhearing. This needs to be a one-to-one conversation with the non-ADHD child or children. They need to be able to ask you questions without hurting the ADHD child.

This is your golden opportunity to make the non-ADHD child feel special, and these are my top six tips:

1. Treat them like a mini adult. Don't sugar-coat or withhold information.

2. Appropriate to age, explain about the child's ADHD behaviour.

3. Let them know which ADHD trait this latest incident will have been linked to.

4. Never, ever lie. Keep it completely truthful.

5. Make it clear that you have to handle the sibling differently, but that this in NO WAY means they are any more special.

6. Ask for their help in getting the best out of the ADHD child. Allow them to feel they are important and have influence in the way things play out in future.

Trust me, this can be done. Not only have I worked with families where previously it has all been going horribly wrong, I've also worked with families where it all then goes brilliantly. And it only takes a few tweaks for this to happen.

It is going to be very useful for the non-ADHD sibling to know that the ADHD child is more than likely going to have ANGER problems, and that these are directly related to their ADHD. The non-ADHD child must not take it personally that the ADHD child will lose their temper on a more regular basis. Instead, they need to know that this is the way the ADHD child's brain works and the very best thing they can do is retreat and take cover! They need to know that engaging with the anger is only going to make the ADHD child worse. If they want the anger to stop, the absolute best thing they can do is move as far away from it as humanly possible. Literally get out of the way of the storm and wait for it to pass.

This goes against the natural tendencies of anybody when they are being screamed at unfairly, but reassure neurotypical children that the ADHD child's brain will be loving the adrenaline arguing brings and is programmed to never give up, will fight to the bitter end and always, ALWAYS, wants to win any argument.

Their ADHD brain will literally keep going on and on and on until it has WON. So let the neurotypical child know they are never going to win and the very best thing to do is to get out of the way. This really will reduce the ADHD child's rage quicker than anything else. The neurotypical child needs to know that WINNING in this situation is removing themselves from it.

If there are two or more ADHD kids in the family then life gets even more challenging. Fairness is key. And I mean fairness in everything, from who sits on the nice sofa longest to who gets to pick the film to see at the cinema. At school, that includes anything that involves choice!

These kids may have different types of ADHD. My own house did: me with my Combined ADHD from my dad, then eleven years later my brother with a different dad inheriting his Inattentive ADHD. Luckily, it was this way round. He was 'my baby' when he was born when I was eleven. He was silent and easy and I adored him. Had the Inattentive one been the older child with a younger Combined sibling it would likely have been a different story.

It is never going to be a bed of roses when you have one or more ADHD children in the house or class. I think getting your head around that and just accepting that knowledge is power (so knowing as much as you possibly can about ADHD children and what their needs are), is always going to make for a more harmonious home and classroom.

It is fairly unusual to have two sorts of ADHD under one roof, but not impossible, as my own case shows. I strongly recommend you learn as much as you can about all three ADHD presentations and what their individual needs are.

Due to their emotional dysregulation and rejection sensitive dysphoria, ADHD children can be having regular emotional outbursts, particularly at the beginning and end of puberty. Remembering that one of the BIG red flags for them is humiliation, the very last thing the neurotypical children need to do is take the mickey or to tease, even in a good-natured way. They need to understand that their sibling/classmate cannot regulate their emotions and some of the displays are going to be quite extreme and shocking. Silence is always the best answer here.

Most ADHD children don't want to be placated or cuddled. They certainly don't want to be told to calm down; they just need to be left to get all their flooding emotions out. And any verbal reasoning you try is going to be met with, 'You just don't understand,' and more than likely a stream of expletives that just cause fresh waves of emotion.

If there is one trait I strongly recommend you educate all kids on, it's the HEIGHTENED SENSE OF JUSTICE. They are going to get very used to the frequent wail of, 'It's not fair,' from the ADHD one, so they need to be aware of where this is coming from. Lack of fairness is at the root of a lot of sibling rivalry. But if you know the rules it is not that difficult to handle. Everything has to be split incredibly fairly. And when I say everything, I mean everything. This particularly relates to screen time and use of devices. If you have children who are sharing devices, then get out your stopwatch and make absolutely sure that everything is split fairly between them. The meltdowns that 'unfairness' cause are just not worth it.

This heightened sense of justice and constant look-out for unfairness will permeate every area of your life. Well, every area that the ADHD child wants. There will be some things that they are very keen not to share. For example, laying the tea-table or doing the washing up. But they are going to fight to the death to make sure they get their fair share of anything their brain sees as pleasure or exciting. This is again where your structure and boundaries need to be in place. They must be rock solid, immovable and non-negotiable. For example, if your structure is that each child gets an hour each evening on the Xbox, it is no good estimating times. You will need a stopwatch, a timer, or definitely something that can't be argued with, so the ADHD child knows for sure it is getting what is fair.

REWARD SYSTEMS

Assuming you are utilising these for the ADHD child, they need to be in place for every other child in the family as well. Please don't make the mistake of only using a reward system for your ADHD child. This gives all the wrong messages to other children. They will see the ADHD child as being rewarded for behaviour they are expected to do anyway. For example, if your system rewards your ADHD child for keeping their bedroom tidy and your neurotypical child is doing this anyway, resentment will soon build.

So jointly put together a reward system with any neurotypical children. A good idea is to use this reward system for them to meet their chosen goals. So for example they might want to complete homework projects by certain dates or commit to netball or singing practice for so many hours a week. Their reward system can be more goal focused than behaviour based, but they definitely need one. Even if they think they don't, I guarantee resentment will build if they see their siblings being rewarded, so encourage other kids to identify goals they want to meet and then reward them. Always make sure these rewards are fair or you'll soon have your ADHD child beating on your door moaning that their rewards aren't as good and IT'S NOT FAIR!

TOP TEACHING TIPS … Don't assume family dynamics will be the same as in families where ADHD isn't present. Don't presume ADHD and non-ADHD siblings need the same kind of teaching or will achieve equally. If you get the fairness bit right, you won't have the sibling rivalry, or not so much of it anyway.

WHAT WORKS BEST … Educate classmates on what is going on in an ADHD child's brain. Open and honest communication about why they exhibit ADHD behaviour is crucial. And make sure reward systems are in place and fair for all siblings. And get yourself the best stopwatch on the market!

*With all the clients I've ever worked with there has only been one exception. This was a young adult living in a part of the world where knowledge of their ADHD would have been seen as a 'mental sickness'.

Although they were diagnosed ADHD as a young child, they did not know they had the condition. The whole family begged me to see this person and it broke my heart having to hear their pleas to understand themselves when I wasn't allowed to tell them that the childhood ADHD diagnosis was the reason they felt and behaved the way they did.

The parents explained to me that if it was known they had ADHD they would never be able to work in the country they lived in: nobody would employ somebody with a mental sickness. I had to respect their wishes and I understood it, but it nearly killed me to do that. It's the only case where I've ever thought it was wise not to be open and honest about a diagnosis.

Important stuff I want to remember:

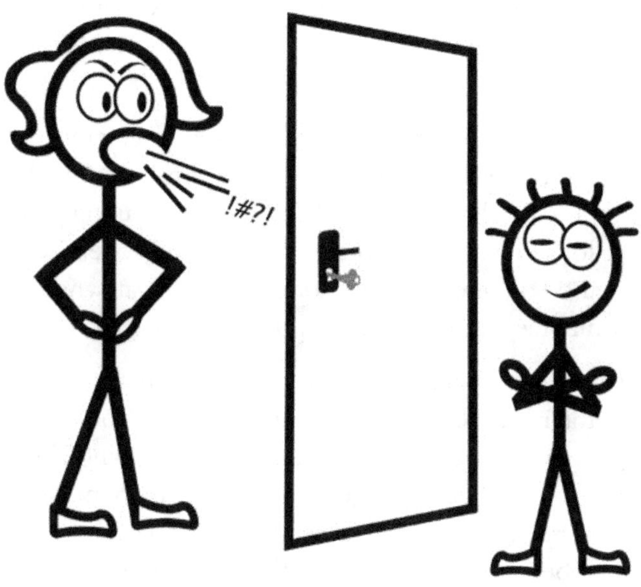

WHEN THEY WON'T COME OUT OF THEIR BEDROOM

Now this is one that definitely will not apply to you at school! But if you have ADHD kids of your own this information could be useful.

Locking themselves away in their bedrooms is typical teenage behaviour but with ADHD there could be a bit more going on. ADHD kids can get VERY frustrated, irritated and angry in their teens. This can be with just about anyone and anything, but particularly brothers, sisters and parents. They can feel anger about a whole host of things, so locking themselves in their bedrooms is sometimes their way of dealing with it.

I'm not talking on an occasional day. This underlying angst, being annoyed about everything, can go on for years. It certainly did for me. From the age of about fourteen I wanted nothing other than to shut my bedroom door and ignore everybody.

Even going downstairs for tea was annoying because I had to listen to other people's boring conversations and answer what I believed to be very stupid questions about my day. I knew what had happened in my day and had no desire to share it with anybody else. Small talk and general chitchat were of no interest to me whatsoever.

I firmly believe the worst thing you can do is force your child to socialise if they are really not up for it and it puts them in a grump. Because a grump can become verbal and lead to shouting and anger and a whole lot of resulting problems. Far better is to let them have their peace and solitude in their room and reappear when they're eighteen or nineteen and in a better, post-puberty, mood!

Don't assume they are doing nothing in their bedrooms. Remember, their busy brains have racing thoughts and keep them very occupied even when they look like they are doing absolutely nothing. Personally, I wouldn't go so far as letting them have their dinner in their room. I've seen this happen and it leads to too much isolation. Far better is to encourage them to come out for their dinner and then to leave them to their own devices.

There are no real rights and wrongs with this one but I definitely wouldn't see it as a problem if your teenager wants to spend an inordinately large amount of time in their bedroom.

DON'T EVEN THINK ABOUT … forcing an ADHD teenager to spend time with the family if they really don't want to. Remember, there is more going on in their head than a neurotypical teenager and, after a busy day at school, they may want nothing more than peace and quiet and their own company.

WHAT WORKS BEST … the times you do see them, make sure you ask them if all is okay and if they need your help in any way. Always ensure that they aren't hiding away for any more worrying reasons. If it really is just because they want to be on their own or their brothers and sisters are annoying the pants off them, leave them to the solitude of their bedroom. Not exchanging pleasantries with Aunt Flo on the sofa or watching *Top Gear* with Dad really isn't going to do them any long-term damage.

Important stuff I want to remember:

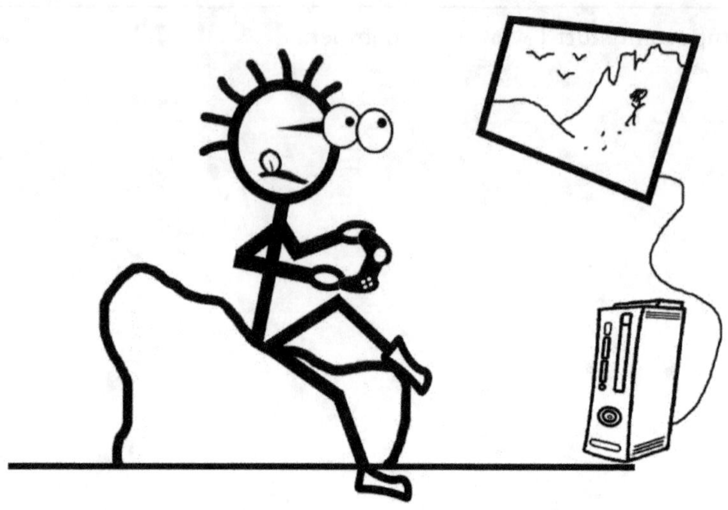

WHEN YOU NEED TO GET THEM OFF GADGETS

I'm sure this is probably way more of a problem at home but it may well also be an issue at some schools, where I'm told a bit of 'freestyle iPad time' can be allowed under special circumstances.

We already know an ADHD child's brain is constantly seeking stimulation. It is never happy 'doing nothing'. It craves stimulation, excitement and for something to be happening – for activity of some sort. Therefore it's easy to see the appeal of electronic devices that provide a constant array of flickering images, changing pictures, vibrant colours and just about everything an ADHD child's brain would kill for. So first off you need to understand what these devices are giving a child. If you're to have any hope of getting them off them, you need first to understand why they are on them.

Normal life can be quite boring for an ADHD child. What is 'enough' for a neurotypical child is soon going to bore an ADHD child rigid. They just aren't going to be able to 'sit nicely' for three hours and read a book. Or concentrate on a film for two hours. It pretty much definitely isn't going to happen unless they're bed-ridden and poorly. They need more; they need activity, drama, different things to look at and LOTS of stimulation.

The fact is, when smart phones were introduced and tablets came on the market all hope of ADHD children being satisfied with reading a book totally evaporated.

Modern technology, in all its shapes and sizes, really does provide the ADHD brain with just what it is looking for. Nothing needs to stay the same! If they are bored with one thing they can, with the flick of a finger, immediately move on to something new. And as everything is bright, shiny and vibrant this can very easily become addictive to an ADHD child's brain. Because when their brain gets a taste for something that feeds it adrenaline, that brain isn't going to give it up lightly. In fact, it is going to fight you to the death for its right to stay stimulated.

So this is what's going on when an eleven-year-old has been on their PlayStation for five hours. Mum may well be climbing the walls knowing that this isn't good for them and they MUST need to move and DO something else. Their brain, however, is having a party and the very last thing it wants to do is to leave that party. Their brain is compulsively pushing them to stay partying and Mum is very much the party pooper.

So now you know what's going on, I can tell you the best ways of dealing with this. If you're reading this before it has become a problem, that's good. If this is already an issue it is going to be more difficult to break habits and patterns of behaviour, but we will come to that in a minute. Let's assume for now this ADHD child has never been near a device and you are ultra-prepared to put a structure and routine in place, set boundaries and introduce reward systems, because it is a combination of these three that will work best. At home this can be as innovative and flexible as you like. At school you might need to put your thinking cap on but I bet there is something you can come up with.

Let's start with structure or routine. Nice and simple, this one. The child needs to know how their day is structured and WHEN it is the time for devices. Every parent and teacher will have their own idea of what is appropriate but let's say, for the sake of argument, you agree they can go on the iPad for an hour in the morning before school and for an hour in the evening. Or at school for thirty minutes of the one-hour lunch break.

If the child KNOWS that in the morning their hour just isn't happening until they are washed, dressed, breakfasted and ready for school, or at school that their thirty minutes does not begin until they've eaten all their lunch, and there is NO leeway on that, this is exactly the sort of structure that will work.

At home they are definitely going to need one structure and routine for the weekdays and one for weekends.

When you've decided this, you need to stick to it. If there's one thing ADHD kids can't stand – and for which they will make mincemeat out of you – it is not sticking to what you've said. An ADHD child will kick against structure and boundaries but it is absolutely what they need to function best. So it is up to Mum or Dad to structure the day in such a way that it works for them, the family and the child and then make sure they stick to it. Do not be lily-livered! Do not be fickle! Don't forget an ADHD child will see through this in seconds and, trust me, you'll regret it.

Any ADHD child, however old they are, needs to be very aware of how their day is structured and this probably means at home you're going to need to have it written up on a black/whiteboard somewhere. Same at school. ADHD kids are time blind and have poor short-term memories, so they won't be remembering exactly what times of the day they are supposed to be doing things. There are numerous ways of making this happen but it is definitely a good idea to have a written schedule for weekdays and weekends, kept where it can be seen by the ADHD child.

Next comes boundaries. Remember, every ADHD child is going to push these because that's what their brain does. Again, you have to have very rigid boundaries. It is no good saying to a child, 'You can have twenty minutes and then your time is up on there,' and then forgetting to do anything about it for forty-five minutes. Or telling them one day that it doesn't matter if they don't have their breakfast before going on the iPad as long as they have it before school. No, no, no! This is the road to ruin. Do not take it.

You need to make it very clear so that the child understands the boundaries. These are going to be different for everybody, but whatever yours are, make it abundantly clear that these are the boundaries and that they are immovable and non-negotiable.

Within these boundaries it is good to give an ADHD child options. ADHD children like to feel in charge, but always remember you are ultimately in charge – although you must try not to make it obvious! For example, you might want to give them the option of having the iPad for one solid hour after dinner or having half an hour after dinner and half an hour after their evening snack. Give the child some options so they FEEL like they're in charge, but always make sure these options fall within YOUR boundaries. If you don't want them on the iPad after 9 p.m., make sure the options are always before 9 p.m.

It's the same at school. If you can give them choices, do. You'll get a much better response if you put them in charge. For example if there are three of them sharing an iPad for an hour, break it down into three 20-minute slots AND put the ADHD child in charge of the timer. I guarantee everyone will get their fair share of time this way.

And now we bring in the parents and teachers of those kids who are already majorly addicted to their devices. They too need to bring in structure and boundaries, but they are going to have a tougher job of it. The way to do this is to negotiate with the child. Speak to them about how much screen time they feel is healthy and have an open debate about what is right for all of you. Not just for them, for the whole family (or class if it's at school). They have to understand and agree what will work best and be FAIR.

Make it a non-judgmental discussion where all opinions are equally valid. Try to encourage the child to see what is sensible, what gives them time to do other things, what gives them enough time to wind down before bed or to get ready before school home-time. Seek their opinion on these things, communicating with them like a mini adult. You'll be surprised how reasonable an ADHD child can be when they are treated like an adult and consulted for their opinion. It's honestly like the flick of a switch. I am putty in somebody's hands if they are nice to me and put me in charge. But the minute anybody starts talking down to me, my attitude is back!

Telling them what to do always brings out the worst. Instead, consult them and ask for their opinion. You might be pleasantly surprised.

You can also agree to try things out. If a teenager thinks it is very reasonable to stay up till 2 a.m. on the PlayStation and insists they won't be tired for school the next day, agree to trial it for a week.

Make a point of asking them at 8 o'clock in the morning how they are feeling. They will inattentively not notice they are shattered, and they certainly aren't going to admit it to you. Saying something along the lines of, 'I hope you're not feeling too tired and have a really good day at school,' (rather than, 'You look wiped out; you shouldn't have stayed up so late, you idiot,') will allow them to realise that it isn't such a bright idea after all – without feeling humiliated.

An ADHD child is always going to need a REASON to come off their device. They are never going to get bored with it, want to do something else or feel it is the sensible thing to do. The easiest way to explain this is that if you are taking away one thing that stimulates the brain, you need to replace it with something else that does the same or similar. You need to give the child something exciting to move onto.

'Exciting' will be different for each child. It could be their favourite TV comedy, dinner, chocolate, milk and cookies in bed or anything that the child would look forward to. That, and only that, is going to get them off their device without a fight.

This is also where reward systems come into play. There's lots more information in the chapter on reward systems but you can use these repeatedly to entice a child off a device.

Just one example could be that if they come off the device at 8:30 p.m. every weekday, without any argument, then on a Saturday night they get to choose the family movie and takeaway. If they fail to do this one night, they lose the choice of movie; if they fail to do it two nights, they lose the takeaway choice as well. The child

NEEDS something like this to entice them. Something has to make it worth coming off that device.

Important stuff I want to remember:

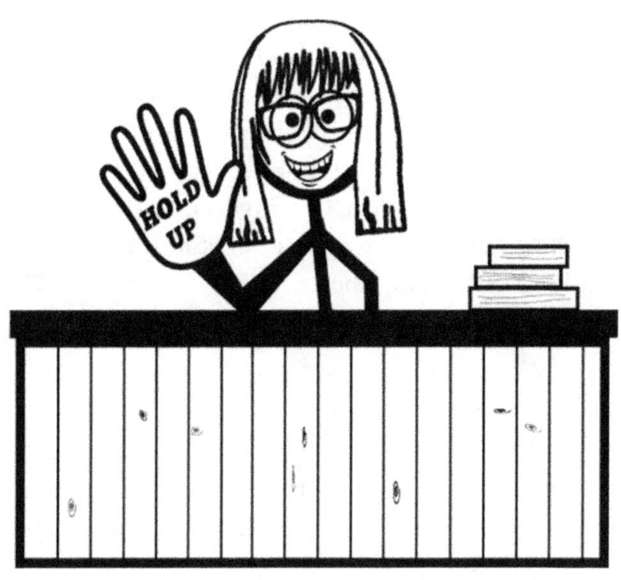

BEFORE I LET YOU GO

And that's it! We are done. This is everything and anything I can think of that will help you understand and manage your ADHD students. But don't feel abandoned! In the 'Where to Find More ADHD Support' section at the end you'll find ways to contact organisations who really do understand ADHD and can offer your ADHD students and their parents more help. You and their families might feel alone, but, I promise you, you absolutely aren't.

Just take a very quick flick back through the pages of this book and remember: an ADHD child is dealing with ALL (or most) of this stuff 24/7. Life isn't easy when you are ADHD, but it can be made a whole lot easier by having parents and teachers who understand what is going on in your busy, fuzzy little ADHD head.

Remember, you are one of the VERY good guys! You are one of the teachers who really wants to understand ADHD kids. I know that because you bought this book. Or maybe you nicked it off somebody! But as long as you've read it, who cares! The intent is the same. There are still some teachers who aren't that interested, who think ADHD kids 'just need to learn to behave the same as all the other kids' and there are some who STILL outrightly don't even think ADHD exists! Ironically, before my own diagnosis, I probably fell largely into that last group. I did think it was just kids who weren't behaving, who hadn't been brought up properly and couldn't control themselves. And there was I stropping around with my attitude and my moderate-to-severe ADHD, completely oblivious! How wrong could I be. But I don't judge anybody for still thinking like that because there is so little education on ADHD, and what it REALLY is, out there.

My one overriding message to you is to remember these ADHD kids are exceptional. Not just special educational needs. Special, pure and simple. Their ADHD brains are going to take them on to be leaders and winners. Yes, that might mean they're a bit more difficult to manage in the classroom but now you understand their brains, hopefully that won't be so much of an issue!

Don't battle them. Don't try to knock the ADHD out of them. Don't try to turn them neurotypical. And don't expect them to be like other kids. They are not. They are different. Yes, they might be a challenge but that's why most of our actors, musicians, comedians, politicians, sports stars, entrepreneurs and probably a good 80–90% of people in the public eye are ADHD.

These kids are driven; they will accept less from you and appear demanding of you and other people around them, but THAT is what drives them on to be leaders and winners in life.

I do appreciate that managing one of those in a class of thirty is a bit of a challenge – but be up for that challenge! Because the odds are that child is going to go on to achieve probably more than the other twenty-nine.

Understand they have no more control over their ADHD brain than the other kids have over their non-ADHD brains. They have just as much right to be their authentic self as all the others.

More than anything I hope I've given you an insight into what is behind ADHD behaviour. Remember, no behaviour just appears. There is always a reason for it. And with ADHD there can be trillions of reasons, and combinations of several traits, which can make it very perplexing for teachers and parents. But please never give up.

Each ADHD child has the potential to be a Sir Richard Branson or a will.i.am, or any one of the millions of very successful ADHD people.

Thank you for being one of the committed teachers who have ploughed through this book, trying to do the best for your ADHD students. I applaud you. And I wish you the absolute best in encouraging these ADHD kids to be successful, confident, ADHD-aware thriving adults who you can look at with pride, knowing you played a part in not only teaching them but in helping them be the very best version of their ADHD selves. My genuine and sincere thanks for caring enough.

Sarah Templeton

August 2022

WHERE TO FIND MORE ADHD SUPPORT

BOOKS

- ## HOW NOT TO MURDER YOUR ADHD KID - INSTEAD LEARN TO BE YOUR CHILD'S OWN ADHD COACH

  by Sarah Templeton
  Gemini Publishing Ltd (2022), ISBN: 9781739958817

  This is the book I initially wrote purely to help counselling clients understand their ADHD kid's brains. Then it went a bit bonkers and started selling round the world! If you are the parent, grandparent or carer of an ADHD child or adolescent, there should be quite a lot of information in this book that will help you.

- ## DELIVERED FROM DISTRACTION

  by Edward M Hallowell MD & John J Ratey MD
  Ballantine Books (2005), ISBN: 9780345442314

  For adolescents/adults with ADHD or wanting to know more about adult ADHD. A brilliant book written by a psychiatrist with ADHD himself. Really easy to read even for those of us who can't concentrate to read books! Funny, incredibly informative and highly recommended. I always say to the teens and adults I work with, 'If you buy only one book on ADHD, make it this one.'

- ## THE ADHD EFFECT ON MARRIAGE

  by Melissa Orlov
  Specialty Press/A.D.D Warehouse (2010)
  ISBN: 9781886941977

  A fabulous book if your relationship is running into trouble because either one or both of you are ADHD. Doesn't just work for married couples. Also brilliant for people in new relationships when one or other is ADHD. Totally helps you understand how the ADHD traits impact on relationships and best ways of rectifying things.

- **TAKING CHARGE OF ADULT ADHD**

By Russell Barkley PhD
The Guildford Press (2010) ISBN: 9781606233382

This is a great book for teenagers and adults alike. Goes into lots of detail about ADHD and importantly gives you lots of different ways of overcoming individual traits. Really easy-to-read book and very useful tips.

- **SMART BUT STUCK**

by Thomas E Brown PhD
Jossey Bass (2014), ISBN: 9781118279281

This is an easy read, with some excellent strategies for children and adolescents who are getting stuck for whatever reason. Purely using case studies of teens he has worked with, it gives different ways of overcoming 'stuckness' from different ADHD traits such as lack of motivation, procrastination, perfectionism, inability to make a decision and more.

CBT USEFUL WEBSITES

- **getselfhelp.co.uk**
- **psychologytools.com**
- **cci.health.wa.gov.au**

AUTHOR'S WEBSITES

- **www.HeadstuffADHDLiberty.co.uk**

For anyone struggling with ADHD and addiction or crime. ADHD psychiatrists, psychotherapists, substance misuse specialists, counsellors, family mediators and a full team to help you overcome any addictions and to guide you through any legal difficulties you find yourself in.

- **www.HeadstuffADHDTherapy.co.uk**

  All diagnosed ADHD qualified counsellors, offering ADHD counselling and coaching to kids, adolescents and adults before, during and after diagnosis. Based in the UK, working internationally with clients worldwide.

- **www.SarahTempleton.org.uk**

  Sarah is a passionate campaigner and fights hard for the rights of ADHD people, and particularly for the rights of children in schools, and adolescents and adults involved in the criminal justice system. An ex-professional actress, she appears regularly on television and radio as an advocate for ADHD understanding and acceptance. All media enquiries should be sent to SarahTempletonMedia@yahoo.com.

GLOSSARY OF TERMS – WHAT DOES THAT MEAN?

ADHD	Attention deficit hyperactivity disorder. Currently diagnosed in three types in the UK:

1) ADHD primarily Hyperactive/Impulsive

2) ADHD primarily Inattentive

3) ADHD Combined – which is by far the largest category.

Anankastic Traits	Similar to OCD but without the negative thoughts attached.
ASC	Autistic spectrum condition. Some prefer this definition to the next …
ASD	Autistic spectrum disorder/Autism
Asperger's	Now classified ASD. You'll see it used still but officially its now high-functioning ASD.
BPD	Borderline personality disorder. Now renamed emotionally unstable personality disorder (EUPD).
Brain Fog	When your ADHD brain can't think clearly. Can be crippling for some, mildly frustrating for others.
CAMHS	Child and Adolescent Mental Health Services. NHS service for children and adolescents up to 18.
CD	Conduct disorder
Comorbidity	A condition existing alongside ADHD. Most common are social anxiety, dyslexia, dyscalculia, dyspraxia, OCD and less common, bipolar and EUPD.
DCD	Developmental coordination disorder – the new name for dyspraxia
DSPS	Delayed sleep phase syndrome. Where your circadian rhythm is approximately four hours behind what would be classified as normal. So natural 'fall asleep time' is 4 a.m. rather than 10–11 p.m.
EHCP	Education, Health and Care Plan
EUPD	Emotionally unstable personality disorder. The new name for borderline personality disorder.
FAS	Fetal alcohol syndrome. Caused when a mother has used alcohol during pregnancy.

GAD	Generalised anxiety disorder
ILP	Individual Learning Plan
NT	Neurotypical. No neurodiversity present.
OCD	Obsessive–Compulsive disorder
ODD	Oppositional defiant disorder
PDA	Pathological demand avoidance
Perfectionism	Striving for flawlessness and setting high performance standards
Psych	Psychiatrist, in this book with ADHD as a speciality
RSD	Rejection sensitive dysphoria
Social Anxiety	A common comorbidity, especially for boys. Usually means being uncomfortable (or unable to be) in crowds, big venues or public transport.
SPD	Sensory processing disorder

WHAT PREVIOUS CLIENTS HAVE SAID ABOUT SARAH

'Sarah literally saved our son's life. School, doctors and CAMHS did not. Without her counselling we would not be where we are today.'

Mum of ADHD Son, 18

'At first I didn't want to see Sarah. I've seen so many rubbish counsellors over the years. But Sarah is totally different. She really understands my ADHD.

My dream has always been to be a footballer, but I'd just been arrested before I saw Sarah and was under investigation. I thought I'd totally ruined my life. Sarah convinced me to still follow my dreams and never give up.

When I was offered a football trial my anxiety made me nearly turn it down, but I asked Sarah if she would come and she did. On a very dark rainy Monday night.

I've now been offered a two-year apprenticeship with a professional football club, which coincided with the week the police dropped their charges. I now feel totally confident and happy within myself and I never did before.'

ADHD Boy, 16

'After ten years being treated for an eating disorder by a very expensive psychologist, it took ONE SESSION for Sarah to realise that my eating issues were due to ADHD and compulsive eating. I'm now finally on the right path to understanding my issues.'

ADHD Lady, 62

'I highly recommend Sarah Templeton and the team at Headstuff ADHD Therapy. Sarah is really passionate about working with ADHD children experiencing difficulties and they all love her.'

ADHD Psychiatrist, London

'My sixteen-year-old son refused to see Sarah at first saying he'd only tell her to 'f**k off' if he didn't like her. She passed the message back through me that he needn't worry, she would tell him exactly the same if she didn't like him!!

This intrigued and impressed him enough to see her and several months of therapy with her later, he now thinks of Sarah as one of his best mates!'

Mum of ADHD/Dyspraxia Boy, 16

'Sarah was not only there for our diagnosed son, she also recognised ADHD in my other son and she has been there for the whole family during our most difficult times.'

Mum of ADHD/ASD Sons, 21 & 17

'It's not until you meet someone who truly understands ADHD that you truly understand yourself. Without Sarah I would still be blaming myself for so many things that I now know can be attributed to my late ADHD diagnosis.'

Steve Lodge, Physiotherapist, High Wycombe

'In our most difficult times, all doors seem to be closed. Sarah's door opened a new world for our son. No words can describe what this meant for us.'

Mother of ADHD Son, 18

'Nothing you can do or say will shock Sarah. She is totally non-judgmental about ADHD and nothing you could say will faze her.

She makes you realise, 'Actually I'm not a complete nutter and my children aren't either.'

It's like a lightbulb moment when you meet and talk to Sarah – suddenly everything you ever did makes sense and you are no longer alone with your own thoughts. She also puts a network of support around you with the adult ADHD support group she set up.'

Louise, 42, High Wycombe

'Sarah worked out in one session that my son's eating problems were connected to ADHD when other professionals hadn't. And at the same time she recognised ADHD in me, his dad. She put us both on the path to assessment, diagnosis and medication and in one fell swoop changed our lives for the better.'

ADHD Dad, 39, and Son, 10

'Sarah could empathise with my ADHD teenage son like no other therapist.'

Mum of ADHD Son, 19

'There is a real lack of therapists who understand ADHD like Sarah does. She is very passionate and amazing at her job and I am not surprised she is so incredibly busy.'

Mum of ADHD/ASD Son, 21

'Sarah's understanding of my ADHD and being totally non-judgmental about my criminal past (which had got me into BIG trouble twice) has made me wish that the rest of our system could be as understanding as her.'

ADHD Boy, 19

'My son struggled all through his teens. He never settled at school. CAMHS wrote him off with 'behavioural problems' until the amazing Sarah Templeton recognised his ADHD and ASD.'

Mum of ADHD/ASD Boy, 23

'I can confidently add 'meeting Sarah Templeton' to my life-changing events! After meeting Sarah I had a whole new perspective on what ADHD means for me and my whole family.'

ADHD Mum, ADHD Sons 13 and 15

'I can't thank you enough. My son has just rung me to say, 'How can someone understand how I tick so quickly? Nobody has ever understood me apart from Sarah.' Thank you. Thank you.'

Mum, Undiagnosed ADHD Son, 37

'I think that letter you read to my son yesterday, from an actual prisoner about how horrific prison is, had a real impact on him. Fingers crossed it stays with him. I would like to write to this lad in prison and thank him. After all he's been through, to think of helping someone else is amazing. I think what you're doing to help keep these ADHD boys out of prison is amazing, too.'

Mum of ADHD Boy, 15

'Sarah, I don't know if you remember my son. We came to you when he had just moved school to do his A levels. Well, I just wanted to let you know that he got THREE A's today!!

The identification by you that he had ADHD (Inattentive subtype) was a turning point and I have no doubt that, had we never come to you, he would never have got these results. The Ritalin allowed him to focus, together with him loving his subjects, the quality of teaching and their ability to build his confidence and belief that he was very capable has all contributed. He has worked very hard these past two years and it has paid off. Thank you!

He has got into the university of his choice to do the subject of his choice. To say we are all thrilled and thankful is an understatement.'

Mum of ADHD Boy, 18

'So many families like ours have been helped by you and your love and support.'

Mum of three, all ADHD, Herts

'I first met Sarah in a Young Offenders' Institute. After a couple of failed attempts at counselling they introduced me to her and I am so thankful they did. She was the first person I found I could talk to and be myself. She was the first person ever to help me to understand that there were reasons for my actions. The first person to ask me how I felt about my mistakes and, if I could, what would I change.

She was also the first person to make me realise that it wasn't too late to have a life – and not just 'get by' but a life that I could be proud of, something that I could build and be proud of.

Despite the fact the prison tried to keep us apart, she kept contact, wrote to me at every prison I was moved to halfway across the country. She visited me at every opportunity she had and kept me calm every time I got angry or could not cope.

Since prison, Sarah has helped me in almost every aspect of my life – she has helped me more than anyone in my life.

Every part of my life since release has been hard till Sarah stepped in. I was just barely keeping myself afloat till she first helped me with a place to live (temporary accommodation and since she has found me somewhere permanent) then set me up in a job so I could work.

Then on top of all that she has now helped me set up in business for myself and got me my ADHD diagnosis. I'm now medicated and confident that in fact I do have a future.

I met Sarah when I was twenty-one; I am now twenty-eight. She is the person who changed my life, the only one to understand, my friend and now I consider her my family.

And above all else the only reason why going to prison was one of best things that happened to me.

If I hadn't have met Sarah I would be back in prison or dead by now. And that is a guarantee.'

Ex-Young Offender, 28, Bucks

Extra notes and reminders: